The Fungus Link to Women's Health Problems

New Insights, New Hope

Doug Kaufmann

Readandlearn LLC
Rockwall, TX

Preface

Without this heart surgery, Annette would surely die. She was wheeled into the holding area, ready for preparation before her surgery when one of her lung doctors walked in and asked what had happened. His office had been notified that she was in the hospital. She could barely speak to him because she was suffocating and her heart was failing. She was told to have this life saving surgery immediately. With that, the lung doctor listened to her lungs and discovered something that the heart doctors may have missed. He quickly asked if they could move her into a minor surgery suite where he performed a quick procedure called a bronchoscopy. A thick white paste blocked her lungs. He tested the paste and found that it was the yeast, *Candida albicans*.

Many doctors are unaware that *Candida albicans* can cause yeast infections outside of the mouth, gastrointestinal or vaginal tract. Fortunately, this doctor knew better. Treatment with anti-fungal drugs and diet prevented a major heart surgery and most likely saved her life.

This is a true story that occurred in Texas. The lung doctor attended a seminar in which I was the keynote speaker two years earlier. Many doctors were in attendance. I spoke on how fungus and yeast (a single cell fungus) mimic very serious health conditions once inside our bodies, including heart disease and cancer, yet our doctors are unaware. As it turns out, inhaling yeast and fungus initiates a chain of events that destroy organs and tissues far from where these organisms enter our bodies. Heart doctors, cancer doctors and endocrine doctors see the end result of yeast and fungal growth and diagnose remote organ failure as the cause when, in fact, the lungs are often the primary organs involved. Yeast and fungi can quickly disseminate from the lungs to other tissues via the blood stream where the heart, by circulating our blood, provides transportation to remote organs that can become infected by these disease-causing germs.

I sat next to this doctor during the seminar, and on Monday morning I received an email from him. Here is an excerpt from that email:

"Good morning, Doug. I want you to know last week and the weekend has changed my life, my practice, and possibly the lives of thousands of people. You are doing fantastic work with scientific validation from very distinguished doctors. What I am now seeing in my patients is the missing link I have been looking for over the last 26 years. I am looking forward to learning and enhancing this relationship to higher and higher levels. Appreciate everything you do!! Best regards..."

I am so thankful that I have been able to teach physicians this lifesaving information. When you teach a patient this lifesaving information, in effect, you have given him a fish, but when you teach a doctor this information, you have taught him to fish. He now finds that he can finally help many of his patients with safe and easy instructions.

I firmly believe that many major diseases can be traced back to yeast and fungus entering the body. What proof exists that fungus plays a role in America's top killing diseases? The #1 cause of death in America is heart disease, and the #2 cause of death in America is cancer. Statin drugs, taken by tens of millions of Americans to lower the risk of cardiovascular events, are anti-fungal drugs. The toenail fungus-killing prescriptive drug, Sporanox, was recently FDA-approved to treat several cancers. Who could refute the correlation between the diseases that we are dying of and fungus? Yet, fungus remains the "elephant" in the examination room!

Will you, the patient, wait until the medical community has finally arrived at that decision (which may take many decades), or will you become proactive now to fend off these tiny, deadly germs from causing tissue changes that mimic the very symptoms that you may be having right now? How does one become proactive in fighting fungus?

Thank you for purchasing this book. Now, roll your sleeves up and let's get to work! We've got a lot of ground to cover!

Doug Kaufmann, 2018

Table of Contents

Foreword
A Note for Your Doctor, from a Doctor Who Has Been There

For patients, this book will open your eyes to the real reasons you have not been feeling well. For doctors, this book gives wonderful insight into the field of mycology, specifically mycotoxicology, and how it impacts the health and well being of many of your patients. My exposure to mycotoxicology was in cases of vaginal yeast infections, toenail fungus and ringworm all too common in outpatient family medicine, and systemic candidemia in intensive care unit (ICU) patients. As a busy family medicine resident physician, the main focus was on the treatment of bacterial infections with antibiotics. Fungal infections, as a potential cause of chronic disease, certainly were not on the horizon for me. It would take several years after graduating from medical school and residency for me to learn the impact of fungus on chronic disease. I gleaned this practice-changing information not from a seminar, but from a patient—someone who came to me for treatment. This patient told me that she saw a gentleman on TV talking about fungus being the cause of a myriad of chronic diseases.

Life moves extremely quickly for a physician; at least, mine does. Getting up at dawn, sometimes having to work through lunch and ending a long day with just a couple of hours with my family before falling asleep from sheer exhaustion was all too common for me. So when this patient strongly encouraged me to watch Doug Kaufmann's TV show, I knew that just was not going to happen. I had never even heard of Doug Kaufmann, and even if I had, I did not have time to listen to him, especially if he was not even a physician. My patient repeatedly sent me links to his show, which I never pursued. Not until about a year later when the same patient reported to me that she had been following the Kaufmann Diet and that she felt so much better, but she would like to feel even better. She wanted a prolonged course of anti-fungal medicines which she wanted me to prescribe.

I knew that if I were going to deny this patient the anti-fungal medication that she was seeking, I would have to give a good reason. She of course sent me links again to the Doug Kaufmann show. I was curious now about how well she felt following his protocol. So this time I clicked on the links, and what I saw made a lot sense. So, I began my own search of the research literature only to find all kinds of information linking the toxic effects of fungus (mycotoxicology) to various chronic diseases, including cancer. Based on my review of the literature, I did prescribe the anti-fungal medicine, and she did experience a higher level of health.

I am so glad I did not forever dismiss what my patient shared with me. The light bulb that lit up in my brain after watching Doug's show is still glowing. Reading his work as well as my own review of the literature reveals that fungal infections, in many cases, present like cancer symptoms and other chronic disorders; accordingly, these may be misdiagnosed. That knowledge has given me the confidence to take a different approach to chronic disease. In one particular case, an anti-fungal regimen resulted in complete resolution of what looked like lymphoma.

Proper fungal diagnosis, treatment and management may be one of the most efficacious and cost-effective game changers in modern medicine.

Christine Salter, MD, DC
St. Louis, Missouri, 2017

CHAPTER 1

There Is Hope!

I dedicate this book to you, one of the millions of very bright, very sick women who feel that you are shackled and muzzled in a doctor's office. Shackled, because you feel immobilized—almost paralyzed—by these mysterious symptoms, and muzzled, because no matter what you say to this, possibly your fourth doctor, it will likely fall on deaf ears.

Once again, blood is drawn. Once again, the same lab tests are ordered. Once again, you find yourself leaving the office without answers, yet once again, writing a $1,700 check. In your misery, you have just enough energy left to wonder, "What just happened?"

You know the drill. You have been through this so many times with so many doctors that this time you took summary notes from the other visits, other tests and other diagnoses. You know exactly the look you will get as you open your notes and begin to summarize the past three doctor visits. On goes the muzzle! You read the recent study that on average, a doctor will listen to you for 11 seconds before he begins offering his input.

You are told that he is a busy man and does not have time to review past visits with you. Rudeness is sometimes contagious in a doctor's office, and if he is rude, his entire staff can be rude too. You are feeling worse with each doctor visit, and to make you even more upset, you have just been handed a prescription for an antidepressant.

To be fair, doctors do not mean to be rude or robotic prescription writers. They simply do not have the answers, and that must be frustrating to them. It would be for me too if I were a physician. No, that does not make you feel any better, but I hope it does open your eyes before making an appointment with doctor number five.

You are smart. Perhaps together, we can figure this out.

I Have Great News for You

I believe I know what ails many women just like you. Thanks to the trust that so many sufferers whom I have had the honor of working with have placed in me, I have been able to prove that my approach has unshackled thousands of women, many of whom felt that they were simply going to die, because doctors had no idea what was causing their health problems. Seeing another doctor or two or three will most likely not resolve your health problems. A Mayo Clinic study showed that 88% of doctor second opinions were either refined from the original diagnosis, or completely different. [1] I would love to tell you that you are in good hands. Please know that sometimes the best hands to be in are often your own, so I'm thrilled about your willingness to learn this new science. I've always loved the idea of partnering a wellness strategy with a doctor you like and who will listen to you.

What You Are Suffering from Is Not Taught in Medical Schools

Over the years, medical schools have become increasingly dependent on drug companies to teach their doctors. Think about it; when you go to a doctor, what does the answer involve the majority of the time? A prescription drug, right? If our bodies suffered from a deficiency of these drugs, then this would be the right approach. However, the vast majority of drugs manage symptoms in ways that might just do more harm than good.

You do not have to take my word for it. Take theirs. The side effects you hear about in the commercials are often worse than the problem you started with. You have heard the litany of potential side effects that go on longer than the commercial itself. Perhaps you have thought, "Now, why would I take that?!" You are not wrong to think like that. Unfortunately, other women do not think like you, and drug sales have skyrocketed since these drug ads hit mainstream TV, radio, magazines and websites.

Never mind that grandma's chicken noodle soup really did cure her family's cold, or that vitamin C cured childhood allergies; that was all yesteryear. Old information cannot possibly be good even if it worked, right? Besides, drug companies can not make ridiculous profits from chicken soup and vitamin C, can they?

We are going to get to the "hope," I promise. I want you to put yourself in your doctors' shoes for just a minute first. Just getting into medical school took so much work that he or she would not risk being ejected by challenging what was being taught. Their natural desires to help hurting people slowly got re-socialized right out of them. Managing disease instead of curing it is so thoroughly ingrained in their training through four years of school plus internship and residency that they practically forget why they became doctors in the first place.

Many have asked about the truly questionable relationships that pharmaceutical companies have with medical schools. How does one take a brilliant 22-year-young brain and convince it that in lieu of fixing a problem, they are to manage it? Quite frankly, I believe that it happens through re-socialization, better known as brainwashing. Those profits we mentioned earlier are all the motivation needed to engage in it. A decade ago, I read of a Harvard Medical School student named Matt who became suspicious when one of his professors began heavily promoting cholesterol lowering statin drugs and belittling any questions as to their side effects. Matt searched this professor's background and soon discovered that he was not only a member of Harvard's staff, but he was also a paid consultant to ten drug companies, including five that sold statin drugs! You may call that a conflict of interest, but I call it blatant cheating. I would love to tell you that such cheating has disappeared from medical schools.

Fortunately, the tide is turning, and I have had the privilege of being a small part of teaching doctors the very things you will learn in this book. To my great joy, they are responding with enthusiasm! As it turns out, many of them did not even like the limitations that managing patients with drugs for 4-6 hours at a time imposed on them. They became doctors to get people better, not to drug them.

My Discovery

After returning from my tour in Vietnam as a U.S. Navy Hospital Corpsman, I found myself sick for the first time in my life. I am not talking about sniffles or flu. I was caught in a cycle of rashes that simply would not end. On top of that, I found myself feeling blue all the time. Instead of the picture of health that I had been, skin eruptions on top of brain and gut problems were now the norm. Oh, there were many other problems that I share in the male counterpart to this book, but I will not bore you with those. I came home from Vietnam with miserable symptoms and no doctor was able to help.

My answer came when I met a doctor who aroused my thinking about this problem from a different perspective. After some library time, I sought prescriptive anti-fungal medication and a radical change from my diet of bologna sandwiches, cookies and beer. (Hey, I was 21 years old!)

As I began introducing vegetables, meats, low-sugar fruits and healthy fats into my diet, my symptoms began to subside. Before too long, I felt like the 19-year-old Doug Kaufmann again. I have since learned that with the exception of the age factor, this is the story of multitudes of people who switch from the Standard American Diet (also known as SAD) to a healthy diet. This diet, however, was different.

At the time, I was doing consulting work at University of Southern California Medical School where Dr. Everett Hughes asked about my strange symptoms. For the next 30 minutes, I told him the odd things that were going on with my health. "Hmmm," he said. "Sounds like a parasite problem!"

BINGO! God knows what worm had gotten into my body, but I did contract malaria while in Vietnam, so perhaps a few tapeworms partnered up with me. I went to the school library a few days later and picked up a book entitled, Parasitology. Man, those worms are ugly! Chapter after chapter taught about how common parasites were in third-world countries and how common infection was.

Then came the chapter that completely shaped my future. As it turns out, yeasts and fungi also parasitize humans. During the monsoon rains, we stayed wet for weeks at a time. When our socks finally came off, so did our skin. Jungle rot, a fungal condition, was common. We all had it. So I know what a skin yeast infection looks and feels like. This chapter proposed that the skin was not the only place that disease-causing fungi grew. Yeasts are single-celled fungi that live harmoniously on and in our bodies, but under the right conditions yeast can become disease-causing as well, similar to other types of fungi.

With the prescription anti-fungals Nizoral and Nystatin in hand, I did feel marginally better, but I would soon learn that medications had severe limitations on my lifestyle, and this same adage holds true today. I often wonder today how many drugs would completely disappear if the people who swallowed them daily only knew that a changed diet, a regular exercise program and the right supplements might do a much better job! My questions at the time were different. How were these fungus-killing drugs working in me? How did fungus enter my body in the first place? Could fungus even be in my brain or causing the low energy symptoms that I felt?

The answers to those questions and more would shape the next 45 years of my career, and tens of thousands of women and men of all ages have seen remarkable turnarounds in their health thanks to the scientific information buried in stacks of medical journals and textbooks. Don't worry; you won't have to read these stacks of journals and books. Nobody wants to do that, not even doctors. Nobody, that is, except me! I have been eager to learn for over four decades, and I am just as eager to share what I have learned with you so that you will know what to do to feel better. Therein lies your hope!

Eat like Your Life Depends on It

In the 1944 book, *The Manual of Clinical Mycology*, written by several Duke University physicians, a few words were dedicated to the necessary change of diet that would have to ensue in order to starve yeast and fungi from your body. You see, fungal cells are very, very similar to human cells, and just as our cells become nourished when we eat, so do theirs. As a matter of fact, without carbohydrates, fungi die. *Remember this throughout this entire book*. If you are one of the millions of improperly diagnosed fungal folks, you must begin to eat what fungus hates to eat! You do not want to nourish disease-causing fungal cells.

Everything I have learned over these years came together packaged as The Kaufmann Lifestyle. The Kaufmann Diet is the very epicenter of this lifestyle. The diet seeks to limit or halt the overgrowth and infection of yeast, fungi and mold in our bodies. The lifestyle is about adopting a whole new way of thinking and being with the purpose of protecting you from yeast, fungi and mold in the first place. Some fungi make poisonous byproducts called *mycotoxins*, which are even deadlier than the fungi themselves. You definitely want to rid yourself of all disease-causing fungi before they begin spewing these poisonous byproducts, and diet is one way of doing that.

If you know how fungi get into your body, what they eat and the conditions under which they thrive, you will know what to *avoid* in order to prevent a fungal infection. Likewise, if you know what keeps them from getting into your body, what kills them if they do and what flushes them out of your system, you will know what to *do* to prevent a fungal infection.

At this point you may be thinking, I don't have a fungal infection; I have PMS, or some other persistent symptoms with a brilliantly thought out name. Please, don't stop reading!

We are learning that fungal infections are behind diseases and conditions far worse than PMS. We now know that there are 5 fungal mycotoxins that possibly cause human cancer, and we know that one of the mycotoxins we are most commonly exposed to in our diets is definitely known to cause human cancer. Worse, our cancer specialists do not know that fungus can cause cancer! If these poisons cause cancer, think of the multitude of other symptoms and diseases they could also cause all the while without doctors knowing about it. Houston, we have a problem!

The Kaufmann Diet can truly be a life-or-death choice for ridding your body of the things that are causing you so many health problems, so do not give up until you have tried my approach for 45 days. You will see that I am asking you to cut out things that you may really love. Impossible, you say? The Kaufmann Diet is far too aggressive, you think? How could this possibly apply to me, you ask?

This is exactly what many of the tens of thousands of daily viewers of my TV show, *Know the Cause*, used to think. It is what the tens of thousands of attendees at my live seminars have said. And it is what doctors that I have had the privilege of mentoring first thought about their patients' health conditions.

And yet, it is totally understandable to think this way *if* you do not know how fungi and their poisons influence every cell in your body.

What if the symptoms you are experiencing were *caused* by yeast, fungus, mold and/or their poisonous mycotoxins? After all, there is a reason you have PMS, or PCOS, or depression, or fibromyalgia or a host of other brilliantly-named illnesses and their symptoms. If you or your physicians do not know that fungi could be causing your symptoms, you could be frustrated and stalled from getting help for years or decades. As a matter of fact, many of you feel exactly this way right now; it is why you purchased this book! You are hoping to finally find truth that can help you.

What I discovered in the early 1970s is that nearly any symptom or disease could have a fungal component to it. While not every one does, the fact that the possibility is left unexplored by physicians means we would be wise to consider a fungal component before labeling the problem unsolved. Just ahead, you will learn about how science has documented this for decades, centuries and even millennia. We have only recently, however, begun to uncover the details and breadth of how fungi can cause common diseases or even mimic them, so do not be hard on your doctors. Clearly, what you will learn is not yet being taught in medical school.

The good news is that just as science has advanced, so have your options in dealing with health issues that have their roots in fungi and mycotoxins. You will not see me talk much about the prescriptions I finally got after coming home from Vietnam. The pharmacies I recommended to the doctors that I worked with 45 years ago had only a small handful of anti-fungal drugs with names like Griseofluvin and Nizoral. Injury to the liver was rare but more likely with these harsh, early generation fungus-killing drugs. Today, not only do we have better prescription anti-fungal options that a growing number of doctors, dentists, PAs and nurse practitioners use, but we also have access to supplement companies who have developed sophisticated, safe, natural and powerful non-prescription products available to anyone.

With all these options, I must recommend that you tell your doctor as you begin this program, because your doctor knows your specific illness and case history, and I do not. The conversation might go something like this:

When did I start coming to you for this problem? Wow! It has been three years already? Although the pills have made life a bit easier, I am a bit concerned about the side effects, and I am wondering if you would help me rule out a germ that I have just learned about as the possible cause of my health problems these past three years. I had no idea that fungi can infect the human body and could off-gas poisons (mycotoxins) that could be making me sick! If you would not mind managing me for the next 60 days, I am going to try an anti-fungal program that will include safe supplements and a diet change. Would that be ok? I will make two appointments with you before I leave today—one in 15 days and another in 60 days—and I will update you on how I am doing during those. Now, can you help me get off of the drug(s) that you have me on?

Some supplement companies invest in research into how plants and animals react to fungi and mycotoxins, and they have discovered a vast array of ways that nature keeps them at bay over time. In many ways, this is the golden age of health options. Today, you will become equipped with knowledge and strategies that not even physicians were regularly exposed to even a few years ago. Many of them still are not. Like many of my viewers and readers, you may find yourself in the position of educating your doctor on how best to treat you. You might even have to give them this book! When a patient with a fungal disorder is helped, it is like giving a man a fish. But when a doctor begins helping more and more of his or her patients because you initiated the idea to think fungus, in effect, you have taught that doctor to fish. His or her patients, in turn, now begin to help so many others!

When I first began this journey, I never dreamed that I would publish in a mainstream medical journal on the fungus link to cancer or regularly be giving lectures to physicians across the country about fungal illnesses. I thought I was the only person in the world who had a fungal problem. My goal was, as yours may now be, simply to get well! But what I have been promoting for over four decades has finally found a place in the wider conversations that women and their healthcare practitioners are having. That makes me proud, but my work is nowhere near being completed.

With each page turned are you finding yourself feeling more hopeful?

You Are Not Alone

Each month there are millions of women who will see yet another doctor or two in a desperate attempt to recover. Therefore, in the upcoming chapters, we will meet women who have been through various diseases and conditions without ever suspecting fungus as the cause. Some of their medical conditions have names given by medical science and some do not. Every one of the women has thought at some point that they may be going crazy or imagining their symptoms, except for the physical evidence of their suffering. Many have been handed antidepressants as a last resort by their doctors who are taught to prescribe. You know the story.

These women are *just like you*. They are your co-workers, your friends, your sisters or your mom. As you read this book, do not be surprised if you get emotional. You may feel hurt or angry as you discover how simple the solutions to some of the world's most baffling ailments can be. You will see that you have known people who died of things that you will learn might have been quite treatable. My staff, associates, friends, family and I are not immune from these feelings and experiences either. We have all lost people very close to us whose suffering and deaths might have been prevented had they only known the link between their food choices and their illnesses, but I would prefer you look forward with hope rather than backwards with regret.

Do not give in to dark thoughts when this happens. Feel the feelings, but do not let them rule you. The knowledge and wisdom you will gain simply was not widely available until very recently, especially in the context of the whole history of medicine. Use those feelings as your motivation to do the things you will need to do to get healthy again. Use them as a motivation to share this message with other people. We cannot change what has already happened, but we can change the future for us, our children and our children's children.

Fungi Are Everywhere

To understand the possible fungal link to your symptoms, you need to know a bit about fungus itself. As we approach this, understand that I realize this is not a pretty flower we are talking about. From the way it looks to the way it smells, fungus is naturally repulsive, and I think that is one of the major reasons why people are resistant to acknowledging it. It seems much less embarrassing to say you have "XYZ disease" than it is to say you have a fungal infection. However, we are going to call it what it is, because your knowledge could mean the difference between comfort and discomfort at best and life and death at worst.

Fungi are found in every ecosystem on planet Earth and quite possibly far beyond. Types of fungi include mushrooms, yeasts, molds, smuts and rusts. They can be found in air, water, soil, indoors, outdoors, within your body and on your skin. Fungi range in size from the tiniest, microscopic spore measuring less than a micron across, to colonies of molds spanning many acres. Simply put, you cannot escape fungi anywhere on Earth. Fungus is ubiquitous.

So, What Good Is It?

Great question! It is easy to feel threatened or even fearful of something that is both repulsive and everywhere, and it is just as easy to think we do not need it. However, fungi play a vital part in the Earth's ecosystem; they are the primary decomposers of the world. Fungi do not process sunlight for energy like plants do, nor do they digest food like animals do. Instead, fungi infest both plants and animals and chemically break them down to produce energy and stay alive.

Ideally, these fungi only infest and break down plants and animals that are already dead. As fungi break dead matter down, they release nutrients into the environment that other plants and animals use to produce energy and stay alive. So you can see that fungi are necessary for perpetuating the cycle of growth, death, decay and reuse that sustains all life on earth. Without fungi, organic matter would merely remain intact, even after the death of an organism, littering the whole world and piling high into the atmosphere. Before very long, plants and animals would have nothing to eat.

Fungi's role as decomposer is not limited it to dead matter however. While many fungi exist within or around other organisms harmlessly, many species of fungi are parasites. This means that fungi can start decomposing you, your pets and some plants while you or they are still alive, working to break down your tissues with the intent of absorbing nutrients necessary to sustain its own existence. Once parasitic and disease-causing fungi have taken root in your body, they will inevitably try to break it down. They cause chemical imbalances inside of your body. Doesn't this sound like what you have been feeling for some time now? Therefore, the only way to stay alive and well is to become actively anti-fungal!

Most plants have natural anti-fungals to protect them, and you will find them recommended on the Kaufmann Diet. Other "plants" are fungus themselves. You will not find these plants on the Kaufmann Diet. If you eat meat, you will do very well on the Kaufmann Diet—if you know which types of plants the sources of your meat are feeding on. Be careful of meat fed fungus-ridden foods, hormones or food contaminated with mycotoxins that mimic hormones like estrogen; instead, gravitate towards meat with anti-fungal benefits. Even if you dislike meat, there are plenty of wonderful protein sources and other foods awaiting you on this diet.

How Many Types of Fungi Are There?

Of the up to 5.1 million fungal species that are thought to possibly exist today on planet earth, 75,000 fungal species have been recognized and categorized. Of those, 300 are known to cause human disease. [2, 3] Simply do the math. This means that another 20,000 or so disease-causing fungi may have yet to be identified. The good news is that whether they have already been discovered or have yet to be discovered, fungi share the need to eat. Whether they are saprophytes, eating dead or decaying material, or parasites living onboard we humans, they thrive in the presence of carbohydrates. Starving them with the Kaufmann Diet may have benefits long before all of the impending diseases caused by these as yet undiscovered fungi are even named!

You are probably familiar with yeasts like *Candida albicans* causing vaginal yeast infections in women. Yeasts are single celled fungi. We will address this in a little more detail in the next chapter. *Candida*, however, is just one of many types of fungi that can detrimentally affect humans. There are a ton of them with ugly names like *Aspergillus*, *Coccidioides*, *Cryptococcus*, *Histoplasma* and *Pneumocystis*. You do not need to know all of their names, however doctors would benefit from knowing them. You just need to know that all of these fungi can affect humans in different ways. They can often cause symptoms in your body that mimic other diseases and can be difficult to diagnose.

What Should You Expect

In this book, you will learn about how to think through your symptoms from a fungal perspective. It is a little different from other philosophies, and there is new terminology you may not be familiar with. We will not go too deep with that, though; we will opt, instead, to offer practical ideas you can implement today.

If you read the book straight through, you will notice a core set of strategies, regardless of the health condition being discussed. That makes sense, given my belief that fungus may be at the center of the many health conditions I cover in this book and many more. There will be certain tactics that differ from each other, but the dietary recommendations will be virtually identical throughout.

I am approaching five decades of helping women just like you, and though there are isolated times when an anti-fungal approach is not called for, I have found it to be an incredibly useful starting point— and endpoint more often than not—for women who are chronically sick and who thought they may never find relief.

Let's get started!

References:
(1) Such, Monica Van, et al. "Extent of Diagnostic Agreement among Medical Referrals." *Journal of Evaluation in Clinical Practice*, vol. 23, no. 4, Apr. 2017, pp. 870–874.
(2) Blackwell, Meredith. "The Fungi: 1, 2, 3 … 5.1 Million Species?" *Botany*, vol. 98, no. 3, 1 Mar. 2011, pp. 426–438., doi.org/10.3732/ajb.1000298.
(3) "Fungal Diseases." *Centers for Disease Control and Prevention*, Centers for Disease Control and Prevention, 1 May 2018, www.cdc.gov/fungal/diseases/index.html.

CHAPTER 2

Digging into Knowledge, Digging out of Sickness

There are three specific ways disease-causing fungi do their dirty work.

First, *fungi themselves* can infect human beings, and when they do, doctors call it a *mycotic infection*. Such infections are well documented throughout scientific literature.

Second, *fungal spores* can affect human beings in a variety of ways. Since fungi are largely immobile, airborne spores are one of the ways fungi spread throughout the natural world. Wind becomes both their friend as well as their taxi. Spores create health hazards in buildings with mold infestations, because they stay inside and circulate as heat or air conditioning allows. It is known that fungal spores can cause and exacerbate allergies and conditions such as asthma or other breathing problems.

Mycotoxins

The third way fungi affect humans could practically fill its own book, which is why I gave it its own heading in this one. Fungi are not the only problems. Their poisonous secondary byproducts, known as mycotoxins, are chemicals that fungi produce as part of their natural life cycle. Fungi produce these byproducts as part of their defense and digestion mechanisms. Different species of fungi produce different types of mycotoxins, many of which harm women in a variety of ways. Clinically, mycotoxins are known to be involved in:

• changes in human genetic material (mutagenic)
• tremors and seizures in humans (tremorgenic)
• cancer in humans (carcinogenic)
• defects to a developing embryo (teratogenic)

- disrupting our hormone-producing (endocrine) system, most notably altering estrogen

Mycotoxins are also known to be poisonous to our:
- DNA (genotoxic)
- nerves (neurotoxic)
- kidneys (nephrotoxic)
- liver (hepatotoxic)
- blood stream, like venomous bites (hemotoxic)
- heart and blood vessels (cardiotoxic)
- lymphatic system (lymphatoxic)
- skin (dermatotoxic)

Finally, mycotoxins can be immunosuppressive, which means they prevent our immune systems from working properly. Basically, they can turn our immunity down or even off.

You see that mycotoxins can have a wide scope of influence on human beings and the symptoms that we have. Now think about your experiences when doctors have told you they do not know what is causing your symptoms. Millions of American patient charts have the words "*unknown etiology*" written in them, because the examining doctor did not know what was causing the symptoms. Once medical schools begin teaching mycology (the study of fungus), this will likely change rapidly.

How Common Are Mycotoxin-Caused Health Problems?
As you have learned, mycotoxins are natural, poisonous byproducts that come from certain fungi. We know that fungi are everywhere. We also know that disease is everywhere. Couple these facts with another fact: medical schools do not teach this information to medical students. You can see why we Americans remain in such poor general health. This book supports the hypothesis that fungi and their mycotoxins cause many of the symptoms and diseases that we are suffering from. Would this not make sense, since our exposure to them is so common and a void exists in the study of mycotoxin-caused illness called mycotoxicoses?

In 1999, The Mayo Clinic published a research paper that discovered the age-old believed cause of chronic sinusitis (a condition that affects about 31 million Americans) was not the bacteria that all patients had been treated for with antibiotics for decades. [1] Rather, a full 96% of these chronic sinusitis patients were found to have fungus in their nasal secretions. Anti-fungal programs (like the Kaufmann Lifestyle that you will read about) would have likely been quite effective for these patients. Unfortunately, even today, doctors continue to treat chronic sinusitis with antibiotics that can fuel fungal infections. Many of our most common health problems may be linked to fungus, not bacteria as is currently thought. Furthermore, as you will learn, the wanton use of prescriptive antibiotics may have dangerous and even life–threatening side effects.

How Fungi Get Inside of Our Bodies

Diet

The acronym for the Standard American Diet is SAD, for a reason. What we eat exposes us to a multitude of fungal organisms and their poisonous byproducts. Fungi are known to contaminate certain crops often because of the conditions in which they are grown; drought and/ or floods can enhance the growth of molds and mycotoxins. The way many foods are stored (in silos) and transported can also play a significant role in their risk for mycotoxin contamination. Most any food is vulnerable to mold growth. You know what happens to fruit like bananas or apples if they are not eaten quickly. Eventually, they grow mold, and we thrown them away. Corn, wheat, peanuts, pistachios and potatoes, though, are among the foods most susceptible to mold and mycotoxin contamination; not coincidentally, they are also staples in many of our diets.

Unfortunately, corn seems to be most vulnerable to fungal growth; it seems to be fungi's favorite food. From scientific studies of all varieties of corn, evidence shows that corn is almost to the point of universal contamination with mycotoxins. Fungi feed on sugar, and if you have ever heard of corn syrup or corn sweeteners, you know that corn contains a lot of sugar. Not surprisingly, where there is an abundance of fungus, there is also an abundance of mycotoxins.

One of the most cancer-causing mycotoxins in the world, aflatoxin, is the byproduct of the *Aspergillus* mold, which has a propensity to grow on corn. [2]

Somewhere along the way, corn was labeled as a vegetable, and we all have had it drummed into our heads that we are supposed to eat our vegetables. However, corn is only a vegetable in the sense that it is not an animal or a mineral. As a food source, it is a grain, and I have been concerned for a long time that all the engineering we have done to corn over the years may have reduced its ability to defend itself against mold growth. I now see gas stations touting the use of the corn derivative, ethanol, in our gasoline. I think that might be the perfect solution for corn. The bad news is that websites like newsok. com and iboats.com are referring to engine gaskets and fuel lines being weakened or broken down by ethanol. If it can do that to engine parts, imagine the havoc that is wreaked inside our bodies when we consume corn derivatives or byproducts like high fructose corn sweeteners (HFCS).

Think about that for a moment. Are you a woman that enjoys a glass of wine occasionally? As it turns out, wine contains ethanol, even though it is not necessarily from a corn source. Ethanol has many sources, but in 2008, over 3 billion bushels of corn produced about 23% of ethanol used in America. As you will learn, ethanol may be best to totally avoid.

Of course, avoiding wine and corn seems not only un-American, but also a slap in the face to America's most popular diets, including the diet that doctors seem to be most in love with—the Mediterranean Diet. Why not have some of America's most popular diets approve of consuming wine and corn? These same diets tout eating mushrooms regularly, too. While I know that some mushrooms may possess medicinal properties, I would prefer to get the same beneficial medicinal effects from other foods or supplements.

First, know that mushrooms are not vegetables. They do not contain fungus; they are fungus. Toxic mushrooms or toadstools produce mycotoxins as well. To this day, there remains controversy about the safety of many mushrooms. According to a 2014 study, there may be about 140,000 species of mushrooms. [3] Approximately 14,000 have been classified and about 7,000 are considered to have varying levels of edibility. More than 2,000 are known to be safe and 700 species are documented to have considerable pharmacological properties. This study concluded with this statement: *"Not only toxic mushrooms, but also some edible mushrooms, contain poisonous compounds, and the severity of intoxication is dependent on the amount consumed."*

In one decade only, from 2004-2014, The World Health Organization has attributed about 346,000 deaths worldwide to mushrooms. [3] In the book, *Defense Against Bioterrorism*, the authors state this about naturally-occurring mushroom poisoning (it is 100% natural for mushrooms to make mycotoxins): *"Naturally occurring toxins include mycotoxins, marine biotoxins, cyanogenic glycosides and toxins occurring in poisonous mushrooms. Staple foods like corn or cereals can contain high levels of mycotoxins, such as aflatoxin and ochratoxin, produced by mould on grain. Long-term exposure can affect the immune system and normal development, or cause cancer."* [4]

Mushrooms are being heavily promoted for their health benefits. Please know that I am not anti-mushroom. Having studied fungal poisons for many years, I am merely questioning whether or not fungi should be eaten at all based on the data presented in this book. Mushrooms are fungi, so consider being prudent in your consumption of them. Unless you are a credentialed mycologist yourself or have a close friend who is one, be careful of pulling mushrooms up from the ground and eating them. Most of the quoted W.H.O. mushroom death statistics occurred in countries where mushroom foraging is common. What are the known benefits of medicinal mushrooms? Can you get those same benefits from other safe sources without eating fungi?

As you continue reading this book, you will better understand why I am concerned that fungus may be the root cause of so much illness and suffering. What time has taught me is that fungus is so easy to avoid contact with if you are aware of your lifestyle and surroundings. This has led me to contend that despite the impeccable and impressive credentials of many in nutritional science, if they do not know fungus, they simply cannot fully comprehend health or nutrition. The Kaufmann Diet makes every effort to minimize fungal and mycotoxin exposure.

While the FDA does limit the permissible amount of one mycotoxin (aflatoxin) in foods, the fact is that many other mycotoxins remain largely unregulated. Given that so many grains like corn and other foods like soy and peanuts are considered staples of the standard American diet, perhaps the safest bet is to assume that any foods containing these ingredients are contaminated with any number of mycotoxins. A quick browse through the ingredients list on the back of many processed food labels will reveal grain, corn and byproducts of both, along with any other number of ingredients that are likely contaminated with mycotoxins. We are commonly eating mycotoxins in our diets, and then both we and our physicians are scratching our heads wondering why we are sick.

You might think, "Surely, the small amounts of mycotoxins in these foods will not hurt me, will they?" In the past few years, science has learned two distinct things about mycotoxins; low-level exposure to them over long periods of time can have the same horrible effects on health as one huge exposure. Additionally, being exposed to several mycotoxins at once is a far greater risk than being exposed to one. Some corn has been found to be contaminated by several mycotoxin-producing fungi. If you are, for example, taking penicillin, regularly drinking alcohol and eating cornbread, your health might be severely compromised simply by doing what we and our doctors believe is normal! Think of a nightclub bouncer letting a few of the wrong people into a club every night, and none of them ever leave. Eventually, there will be enough of them to cause whatever trouble they want. In that club, the owner could see what is happening and put a stop to it. In our bodies, these troublemakers are microscopic, making fungi and their mycotoxins difficult to discern as the root cause of any health problem. Just as no bouncer in the world can prevent what he cannot see, so also is no doctor able to diagnose what he cannot see.

Consider also that physicians who are beginning to learn of the health problems associated with mycotoxins are discovering that the immuno-compromised patient is the most vulnerable to fungal diseases. While it is obvious that those without an immune system are most vulnerable to any disease, keep in mind that fungal mycotoxins themselves cause declining immunity. So, if you are inhaling mold or eating mycotoxins daily in your food, you can see how you might end up with lowered immunity, a condition that scientists call being immunocompromised.

Furthermore, many newer studies today report of fungal illnesses affecting the immunocompetent rather than the immunocompromised. This is predictable, because before fungi negatively impact your immune system, you are immunocompetent! The problem remains that the accurate diagnosis of a mold-related health problem requires knowledge that most healthcare providers simply do not currently have, because medical schools have yet to accept the prevalence and seriousness of mold-induced health problems. Medicine is slow to change, so you must not be. Are you willing to wait until this is finally accepted and taught in medial schools, knowing that this will likely take decades?

The Air We Breathe
I stated above that if you are inhaling mold regularly, it might be compromising your immune system. Fungi and especially mycotoxins are *microbial*, which means that they exist on the microscopic level, just like viruses and bacteria do. That means that they can catch a ride on the movement of air, even indoors. Ironically, some of our more modern, efficient and largely airtight construction techniques make buildings more susceptible to fungal contamination than they were 50 years ago. It is not uncommon for spaces to appear remarkably clean, yet they could still harbor some sort of hidden fungal organism. Those microbes get into the air, and we inhale them into our lungs.

This is where we can run into severe problems. Some of these inhaled molds make us hack and cough for months, and we find no relief in doctors offices. Then one day, the cough is diagnosed as lung cancer by a CT scan.

After learning the bad news, the first question that pops into your head is, "Are those scans accurate?"

"Of course, they are highly accurate at pinpointing lung masses," your doctor states.

He is absolutely correct! But lung masses are not necessarily lung cancer. Testing far beyond a scan is required to diagnose or rule out a fungal cause of the mass. Lumps are not necessarily cancer. Inhaled mold can look for all intents and purposes exactly like many respiratory conditions, including asthma and even lung cancer. (We go deeply into the topic of cancer later in this book.)

Fungi prefer dark, damp places, so they lurk in dark corners, ducting, insulation and behind walls. This is especially true in homes or buildings that have experienced flooding, broken pipes or some other sort of water damage. Fungal colonies can proliferate through many types of building materials including drywall or even the structural wood that built the home. Wood's strength comes from linked sugar molecules called cellulose, so if it ever rained on the wood that eventually built your home, even while still at the lumberyard, you could have a moldy home. Many homes that were rained upon while in the process of being built are vulnerable to fungal growth; fungi can impregnate the wood and then eat the cellulose for survival. While remediation is possible, it often means discarding the affected material often at huge expense.

Remember that fungi are generally immobile. The primary exceptions to this rule are fungal spores which employ a method of reproduction similar to that of a dandelion. These spores can become airborne, and when they do, they can contaminate indoor spaces. This process has been identified as making allergies and asthma much worse for those who suffer with them.

But can inhaled mold cause more than sneezes and sniffles? Indeed, it can! A study from 2013 showed that 27 patients misdiagnosed with lung cancer were actually found to have lung fungal infections. Fungi or fungal spores had found their way into these patient's lungs and grew to the point that they looked exactly like (and were actually di-agnosed as) cancer tumors. [5]

Fungal contamination of buildings is a known cause of Sick Building Syndrome or Toxic Building Syndrome. Often, these problems are swept under the mat in large part, I suspect, by insurance companies who are unwilling to pay for remediation or resulting damages. Can-didly, I do not blame them, since most every home that has ever had water damage likely has a mold problem and might require some form of remediation. What insurance company wants to empty their bank accounts to rebuild 80% of American homes? This I under-stand, but concealing the health problems caused by sick buildings is undeniably wrong.

This "moldy home" phenomenon was unknown until about 25 years ago. Today, many landlords include clauses in rental contracts indem-nifying themselves against legal action pertaining to mold, mildew and any subsequent health problems they cause. Despite this and the many mainstream medical professionals insisting that indoor mold, mildew and other types of fungi can only cause superficial problems like sniffles or sneezing, there is a mounting body of evi-dence to the contrary. Furthermore, the personal accounts of people who have lived in or dealt with moldy homes or buildings testify to the highly toxic effects of mold and mycotoxins. We are in our infancy of understanding and recognizing the damage being done to our organs by inhaling toxic mold inside our homes or other buildings.

Skin

Many species of fungi, known as dermatophytes, can live on our skin. You are likely familiar with these. The most common types of fungal infections of the skin include athlete's foot, ringworm and jock itch. These are usually treated with over-the-counter medications. Cracks or folds in the skin or "pendulum tissues" can provide an access point for opportunistic yeasts and fungi, since dampness and heat occur directly underneath these tissues. People who work in the outdoors (particularly those whose work involves soil) are regularly exposed to fungi, and their skin can become infected by these organisms.

There is a reason why doctors regularly prescribe medications or suggest over-the-counter remedies for fungal infections of the skin. The proof that it is harming you is right there in front of their eyes; they see the harm fungus is causing you. If they could only peer inside of your lungs or perhaps other parts of your body it would look just as bad—swollen and irritated. But inside of us is invisible to them, and routine office visits offer complaints but rarely a fungal diagnosis unless it can be seen.

Know that not every skin problem is due to fungus, but if you have a skin problem that is resistant to traditional treatments of cortisone or other topical medications, ask your doctor if he would mind doing a KOH test on the affected skin. This is a skin fungus test, and within 30 minutes the results are usually available to you. Not all doctors are equipped to do this test.

Dermatophytes are not the only skin contact fungal diseases of which we must be knowledgeable. Indeed, skin contact with fungi will likely lead most of us to a dermatologist. Many procedures, tests and medications may follow, all in their sincere effort to accurately diagnose and fix your skin problem. But as a 2017 research paper in a respected medical journal stated, "Cutaneous implantation and systemic mycoses are neglected diseases that affect millions of individuals worldwide." [6] Once your skin is "implanted" with fungus, finding a dermatologist who is competent in recognizing fungal infections is difficult. Always ask if you can try the anti-fungal program as outlined in this book. Relief may soon be yours. We will talk in detail about skin fungal conditions later in this book.

Intimacy

There is growing evidence to support the supposition that two people involved in a sexual relationship can pass fungi back and forth between each other, subsequently producing symptoms in themselves and their partner. The yeast *Candida albicans* not only causes vaginal yeast infections but is also the most common fungus involved in male prostatitis. [7] As we just learned, many fungi are dermatophytes, meaning they live on the skin. As a natural part of an intimate relationship, these organisms can pass between sexual partners. This idea expands our perception of sexually transmitted disease, and it will be more thoroughly covered as we progress in this book.

Antibiotics

In his book, *The Genus Penicillium*, Dr. John Pitt wrote, "It is ironical that this humble fungus, hailed as a benefactor of mankind, may, by its very success prove to be a deciding factor in the decline of the present civilization." [8] While Dr. Pitt perhaps was not speaking necessarily of the side effects associated with antibiotics, he most likely did not realize the prophecy of his own words.

If you remember anything from ninth grade biology, you may recall the story of the discovery of antibiotics that was credited to Dr. Alexander Fleming. Like many advances in science, his discovery was serendipitous, an accidental discovery. In his lab, Dr. Fleming's petri dishes became contaminated with mold that had been growing on an orange. He realized that bacteria would not grow around mold colonies in petri dishes.

Fast forward many years later. Dr. Fleming isolated what would become known as penicillin—the first antibiotic—from the *Penicillium* mold. The medicine that would in a very real way alter the course of humanity by saving millions of lives was a fungal metabolite (or as you have come to know it in this chapter, a mycotoxin). While antibiotics have advanced far beyond what Dr. Fleming initially discovered, what remains is this: *A drug that is essentially a mold poison is still one of the most commonly prescribed medicines today.*

Antibiotics are so overused today that I believe when people have too much mold in their bodies already and are prescribed yet another antibiotic, we inappropriately refer to their sometimes life threatening symptoms as being "allergic" to penicillin. Millions of Americans are allergic to penicillin; or are they? It is not uncommon to find *Penicillium* mold contamination in homes and other buildings. Perhaps many of those diagnosed with penicillin allergy may be living in a home that is filled with *Penicillium* fungus, and they are constantly inhaling and being filled with this mold. If so, it is conceivable that one tiny peni-cillin pill could push them over a "mold threshold," thereby causing a very dangerous life threatening allergic reaction called anaphylaxis.

Antibiotics are clearly among the most groundbreaking achievements in medicine, and there is no doubt that they have saved many millions of lives. However, the darker side of antibiotic use and abuse has only started to be uncovered in recent years. The most glaring example of the potential dangers associated with antibiotics has been the rise of antibiotic-resistant bacteria such as MRSA and other so-called super-bugs. These deadly bacteria are the result of the overuse and misuse of antibiotics researchers tell us. Since we cannot get antibiotics with-out a prescription, in my opinion, blame should be placed directly on medical schools.

As scary as antibiotic-resistant bacteria are, they are not the only problems associated with the overuse of antibiotics. Many diseases and conditions are now being linked to the medicine once thought of as humanity's silver bullet. Excessive antibiotic use has now been linked to the incidence of breast cancer and other types of cancer. [9] More recently, the antibiotic Amoxicillin, perhaps used by every par-ent in the world, had its use linked to hyperactivity in children. One wellness website states that Amoxicillin sometimes causes behavior-al changes, including, "…hyperactivity, (and) agitation…" [10]

So what we see as a fungal–mycotoxin link to breast cancer, hyper-activity or any number of symptoms or diseases leaves our doctors and researchers scratching their heads trying to figure out the cause, when all the while, the cure and the cause might have very well been one and the same.

An antibiotic's job is to kill bacteria, and they are very good at it. When doctors first began prescribing antibiotics, everyone from the manufacturers to the pharmacists and doctors to the FDA overseeing it all thought that these drugs just killed pathogenic (disease-caus-ing) bacteria. A few decades ago, however, a relevant discovery was made in medicine; little did we know that the body was loaded with good bacteria. It covered our skin and made up a good chunk of our immune system in our intestines. But doctors had been killing these good and essential bacteria with antibiotics since the 1940s, leaving most brilliant researchers wondering why Americans were plagued with gut problems!

You see, antibiotics do not know the difference between disease-causing, bad bacteria and the beneficial bacteria that we need to be healthy. So, we all became unhealthy until the word *mycotoxin* was developed. We then understood that our best selling drug was a fungal poison. Antibiotics were and still are indiscriminate bacteria killers (kill good and bad bacteria), and we had better learn how to restore the good bacteria in our guts before it is too late.

The internal flora, this beneficial bacteria that we all have in our digestive tracts, helps keep our bodies healthy and in balance. Science has only recently begun to understand the role that the over two pounds of bacteria living in every human being plays in health. These bacteria aid in the digestion of food, production of energy, immunity and manufacture certain nutrients. Their presence is entirely natural, and their relationship to us is symbiotic, which means that we can both live together in harmony. The more we learn about these bacteria, the more the importance of their role in health seems to come into focus. One can see how 70 years of indiscriminately killing them with antibiotics might lead to ill health in large numbers of people.

While sometimes necessary, antibiotics can disrupt these beneficial bacteria. We all have *Candida* yeast in our guts, but using antibiotics can lead to yeast overgrowth in the gut. With beneficial bacteria no longer maintaining balance in the terrain of the gut, pathogenic (disease-causing) yeasts can flourish. For many, this is the first step towards a systemic fungal problem, or a problem that attacks your entire body.

Often, the problems associated with systemic fungal infections can be difficult to diagnose, and unless your physician understands the role yeasts can play and the subsequent problems they can cause, a fungal problem will likely go undiagnosed. For this reason, antibiotics should always be considered a remedy of last resort. However, all of us know that most doctors reach for antibiotics first, and at this point in the state of medical training, many of them do not learn about any other options.

Local vs. Systemic Fungal Infections

Many mainstream health practitioners will say that fungal infections are merely local infections except for in the most immunocompromised of patients. These types of local infections including ringworm, toenail fungus (onychomycosis), jock itch and vaginal yeast infections are sometimes caused by dermatophyte fungi that are nourished by our keratin (a substance forming the chief constituent in the hair, nails and horns of animals). These infections are regarded as annoying but otherwise superficial problems. Generally, the culprit is assumed to be nothing other than damp socks or clothing, a cat scratch or something that is usually not deeply harmful, and the infections are often treated with over-the-counter creams, or at most a one-time, one-pill prescription for an anti-fungal drug.

However, some practitioners have noted that if you have a fungal condition anywhere on your body, it *could* be a sign of a deeper, more systemic fungal problem. Lynn Jennings, M.D., who has provided us with many of the case studies you will read in the book, has frequently said in numerous articles that if you have any sign of a fungal infection, you likely have yeast overgrowth in your gut. From the gut, yeast can spread throughout the body.

Common Yeast Infections: A Sign of Something Worse

Doctors know that *Candida albicans* yeast is a single cell fungus, know it can be disease-causing and know how to treat it. Yeast infections are annoying, uncomfortable and more than a little embarrassing. The fact that nearly every woman has at least one at some point in her life is no comfort.

You have tried all the over-the-counter medications. The 7-day treatment. The 5-day treatment. And thank God for the 1-day treatment when it works. Still, you would rather not have to keep going back to the store, hoping no one sees you grab the tube off the shelf, buying

14 other things you do not really need just so you can get some relief, praying that the cashier does not notice with an awkward glance what you have hidden in among the other items on the conveyer belt, and finally beseeching the throne of heaven that there will be no price problems with that product that will cause your well meaning cashier to yell halfway across the front of the store to her manager. Whether you have been there or just have an active imagination around a well-founded fear, you know what I am talking about. And you are ready to *quit* talking about it.

With all our knowledge about yeast infections, few know that yeast infections are often intensely related to other diseases. Our familiarity with yeast leads many of us to separate it mentally from the unfamiliar varieties of fungus and mycotoxins that have strange-sounding names. That familiarity extends beyond our knowledge of yeast from a medical perspective. We know yeast as a normal part of a class of food so important that we often equate it with life itself.

Yeast Is Not Always Our Friend

Have you ever wondered why a yeast infection is bad while yeast in bread is considered good? The way most people talk about it, we are led to believe that there is somehow a difference between the two. There are indeed different species of yeast; however, all of them do the same thing all fungi do. As they feed on the sugars in grain, they off-gas, and this is exactly what makes bread rise. It is also what makes you bloated when you have a yeast infection.

You might hear this and think, "Yeah, but cooking bread kills yeast, right? After it does its job in the bread, it's not going to hurt me."

I have got news for you. Fungi are not like bacteria and viruses, which must have very specific environments to survive. Remember the job of fungus: Fungi either break down dead stuff or parasitize animals. Fungi have to be able to thrive in any environment, good or bad. This includes a healthy human intestine or within the Soviet Chernobyl Nuclear Power Plant, site of the 1986 nuclear accident. What could possibly be living there? The same fungi that can survive in any environment in the world.

Even when fungi are destroyed by heat, their mycotoxins are not, because they are heat stable. When you cook rice or pasta, the boiling water can rid the grain of fungi, but if those fungi have already deposited their poisonous mycotoxins within that food, you are going to eat them! Some studies suggest that it is impossible to get rid of mycotoxins once deposited. This means fire or even autoclaving food will never render it mycotoxin free. Therefore, mycotoxins remain in your bread and other yeast-containing baked goods long after they come out of the oven.

You might have read about nutritional yeast being a healthy food. Nutritional yeast is a deactivated species of yeast known as *Saccharomyces cerevisiae*. You've seen this word before. This is the same type of yeast used to make bread and beer. Heat is used to deactivate the yeast. This is an exciting yeast, as yeast goes, in that scientists are finding that it has the potential to reduce mycotoxin toxicity in agricultural settings. However, given the message in this book, I would be cautious of eating any yeast or fungus until scientists are able to better understand (and publish) their ability, or lack thereof, to cause human health problems.

If you have an irritating condition like PMS or migraines, think back to before you started seeing symptoms. Did you also have a yeast infection? Most likely the answer is, "Yes. I have had cycles of them over and over." I heard so many stories like this when I worked in clinical nutrition. Resolving health problems is very much like puzzle building; some are easier than others, but once assembly starts, all that is required is time to figure it out!

I am certainly no wizard. People who have earned their degrees in fungal studies are called mycologists. There are actually very few non-mycologist people like me in the field of mycology, or the study of fungi. This is a very complicated field, but I have studied the link between fungi and human symptoms and diseases for decades. This is why I called my TV show and website *Know the Cause*. The cause is so often fungus!

What about critically serious health conditions like autoimmune disorders or cancer? A yeast infection could not possibly be related to these diseases and conditions, could it? For decades, the results of many peer-reviewed studies have shown this could have been the case, and the evidence continues to mount. Perhaps this is the very reason that our brightest and best brains have failed to resolve any disease process! Not learning mycology in medical training leaves a void that is impossible to fill.

You will see yeast infections mentioned again and again in this book. That is because, unbeknownst to most women and many physicians, yeast infections transcend the vaginal tract. As a matter of fact, over 40 years ago, The Journal of The American Medical Association published an article that confirmed that when a woman has recurrent vaginal *Candida* yeast infections, it is important for the doctor to know that yeast in her intestines must be rid along with the yeast in her vaginal tract! [11] So many women see an OB-GYN one day for a chronic vaginal yeast infections and a gastroenterologist the following day for stomach and intestinal problems, when all the while, the OB-GYN might have cleared both problems if she knew of this important paper. When you have more than one yeast infection, especially in a short time, your guard should go up. It might be time for you to follow the Kaufmann Lifestyle before things get worse.

I hope you can see now how important it really is to know what causes the problems you have had that led you to pick up this book. I am glad you did, and I do not believe it was an accident. You are receiving this knowledge because you need it. You have been laboring under the heavy burdens of not knowing what is causing your problems, finding no one who can help you identify them, which leads inevitably to having no idea how to treat them. The roulette wheel of drugs to try has probably left you feeling worse than when you were just dealing with your symptoms.

The good news is that you are now more knowledgable about fungus than many doctors just because you read this far. You know better now than you did when you picked up this book what may be causing your health problems, and whether you realize it or not, you now know better what to do about them. Female intuition is a wonderful thing!

References:
(1) Ponikau, Jens U., et al. "The Diagnosis and Incidence of Allergic Fungal Sinusitis." *Mayo Clinic Proceedings*, vol. 74, no. 9, 1999, pp. 877–884., doi:10.4065/74.9.877.
(2) "Aflatoxins." *National Cancer Institute*, www.cancer.gov/about-cancer/causes-prevention/risk/substances/aflatoxins.
(3) Jo, Woo-Sik, et al. "Toxicological Profiles of Poisonous, Edible, and Medicinal Mushrooms." *Mycobiology*, vol. 42, no. 3, 2014, pp. 215–220., doi:10.5941/myco.2014.42.3.215.
(4) Radosavljevic, Vladan, et al. *Defence Against Bioterrorism: Methods for Prevention and Control*. Springer Netherlands, 2018.
(5) Guimarães, Marcos Duarte, et al. "Fungal Infection Mimicking Pulmonary Malignancy: Clinical and Radiological Characteristics." *Lung*, vol. 191, no. 6, 2013, pp. 655–662., doi:10.1007/s00408-013-9506-0.
(6) Queiroz-Telles, Flavio, et al. "Neglected Endemic Mycoses." *The Lancet Infectious Diseases*, vol. 17, no. 11, 2017, doi:10.1016/s1473-3099(17)30306-7.
(7) Kibbler, C. C., et al. *Principles and Practice of Clinical Mycology*. Wiley, 2005.
(8) Pitt, John I. *The Genus Penicillium and Its Teleomorphic States Eupenicillium and Talaromyces*. Academic Press, 1979.
(9) Dobson, R. "Antibiotics May Be Linked to Risk of Cancer." *Bmj*, vol. 337, no. aug21 3, 2008, doi:10.1136/bmj.a1381.
(10) Iannelli, Vincent. "Amoxil Can Treat Infections in Children." Verywell Health, *Verywellhealth*, www.verywellhealth.com/amoxil-description-side-effects-of-antibiotic-2633173?_ga=2.228288541.1283684324.1534285467-1841237655.1534285467.
(11) Miles, Mary Ryan. "Recurrent Vaginal Candidiasis." *Jama*, vol. 238, no. 17, 1977, p. 1836., doi:10.1001/jama.1977.03280180040023.

CHAPTER 3

Sexual Intimacy and Fungus

Throughout the years, I have spoken at various events across the US. The crowds varied from 15 local customers at a health food store to thousands of people crowded into arenas. On occasion, I also teach continuing education for doctors, so I can spread the knowledge I have gained to those in the best position to do something with it. Wherever I speak, there is one topic that almost everyone wants to hear about, yet no one seems to bring up.

I am not afraid to be the one to bring it up.

I must, because it dovetails so perfectly with my topic. If you have ever had a skin disease on or near your genitals or an inflammation of your sexual organs, you know how uncomfortable it can be physically, emotionally and socially. It is painful and embarrassing. When it is a recurring condition, it begins to feel like you are living under a cloud that never stops raining. You withdraw from others, and if you are married, this includes your husband. Without intimacy—emotional or sexual—you feel as though your relationship with your husband withers and dies. If you are like most people, you are not talking about it, and your husband may think there is something wrong with him, or at least think that *you* think there is something wrong with him. Obviously, this is not a recipe for a healthy relationship.

To say that an illness affecting your sexuality is much more than a physical ailment is to tell you something you know all too well. Or do you? So many women suffer from illnesses that their doctors simply do not know the cause of. Few physicians understand that sometimes the answers to your questions and concerns lie in the fact that certain germs known to cause human illness can be passed back and forth on the skin. Unfortunately, this is a relatively new understanding.

Most of our physicians were not privy to that information in medical training simply because their teachers were not either.

I can tell you there is hope and healing available for your body. Healing your relationship may require more, but God willing, let us try to help you get rid of your physical disease forever.

Truth You May Not Want to Hear

Diseases on or in sexual organs that are not genetically driven are often transmitted sexually. Therefore, not only do they become a lifestyle problem, but the root of them may have been your lifestyle. For many, the 1960s changed everything, sexually speaking. In the 1960s, the average teenager learned of sexual mores or norms in magazine ads, TV shows, movies and songs. If we could not be with the one we loved, so the song went, we were supposed to love the one we were with. We did. We learned that if it felt good, it was OK to do. Little did we understand what the ramifications of our actions would be 50 years later. But even those who did not live in the 1960s still have this personal problem that our close friends and doctors have no idea how to successfully treat.

The purpose of this book is not to dish up regrets. Rather, it is to teach you. You see, our escapades then might just be responsible for our health problems today. In the 1960s—and to a certain extent even today—our knowledge of sexually transmitted diseases was fairly limited to gonorrhea and syphilis, each treatable with a dose of antibiotics. It seems that those antibiotics successfully treated many cases of sexually transmitted diseases, but unfortunately, today some of them are back with a vengeance. Women and their partners must be vigilant, because sexually transmitted diseases (STDs) continue to grow in numbers. While syphilis and gonorrhea are still causing many sexually transmitted health problems, genital herpes, human papilloma virus (HPV), hepatitis B and chlamydia are some of the most recognized sexually transmitted diseases in America today. And there are many others!

Germs, in particular fungal germs, may play a role in some of these diseases. As you now know, this book is filled with brand new information about the relationship between fungal poisons called mycotoxins and their ability to cause illness or diseases. Yes, fungi can be transmitted between loving couples. Is fungus causing your health problems? Let's study this a bit more.

First, know that fungus can be sexually transmitted and might lie dormant for a long, long time. Scientists know that fungi can live inside our bodies as symbionts, where both we and parasitic fungi can live in harmony. We all have *Candida albicans* inside of us, yet it is not problematic until it inadvertently activates as a pathogen (symptom or disease inducer). Because so few physicians understand the role of fungus inside our bodies, this has been greatly overlooked. Recall that fungus requires transportation to become mobile. When it is the cause of a disease or multiple diseases, it must gain access to the affected organs and systems somehow. Sex is one of the ways it gains access.

There are two things that happen during sex that create an opportunity for fungus: A lot of frictional skin-to-skin contact takes place along with an exchange of fluids. We talked in the last chapter about fungi that live on the skin, but know that since fungi are everywhere, both male and female fluids exchanged during sex can be infested with yeast and fungi as well. Just as bacteria can cause bladder infections, so can yeast and fungi. Remember, it is called a "yeast infection" for a reason! Fungi and yeast have also been isolated from semen, so it is likely that males do play a role in some women's yeast infections. According to the Mayo Clinic, yeast infection can occur in men, causing swelling of the penis, a condition called balanitis.

It is really a simple numbers game; the more people you have sex with, the more sexually transmitted germs (including fungi) you are potentially exposed to. As you will soon see, there is enough risk with just one partner to require active management of that risk. When you add in multiple partners, the risks are not merely added; they are multiplied because of the partners they were previously with. But throughout this chapter, know that you also have an incredible immune system that normally rids the body of disease-causing germs, whether on the skin or in our fluids. Do not think that the past has somehow come back to haunt you, because the younger you were, the stronger your immune system was. Rather, this chapter helps you understand that sometimes, the symptoms and germs you may now be dealing with just might have been dormant for decades! Age plays cruel tricks, one of which is to make us more vulnerable to germs. Again, being actively anti-fungal can help no matter what age you are!

Are We Passing This Back and Forth?

In the last chapter, we talked about chronic yeast infections. Many women experience yeast infections that go away only to come roaring back after a few weeks or a few months. Traditionally, your doctor treats yeast infections in the vagina. As you have learned, the vagina is a reservoir for yeast to grow in, but the gut can harbor that yeast and keep the vagina well supplied. It is a vicious cycle unless and until doctors realize that in many women, vaginal yeast infections will continue until the gut yeast is also killed. Elimination of gut yeast overgrowth is often necessary to successfully treat the chronic vaginal yeast condition. Sometimes it is not the gut's fault, but the skins fault. But sometimes, it's not even your skin!

During sex, contact occurs in a number of ways through which these microscopic fungal cells can gain access to our bodies: skin on a hand, in a mouth or anywhere else that human skin touches human skin. If one person who has a pathogenic yeast on their skin rubs against one who does not, it only stands to reason they could very well pass yeast where it had not been before. During a normal, healthy and loving sexual relationship, these skin fungi can transmit fungus back and forth. As you continue reading, you will learn that some yeasts grow on our skin.

During my many years of working in clinical nutrition alongside physicians, I have worked with many women who openly spoke of their personal struggles with chronic yeast infections, hoping nutrition had something to do with them. Many asked their gynecologists if these infections might have anything to do with their male partners. Gynecologists, more than most doctors, know what fungus is because they see yeast infections all the time. Yet most are not trained to consider any link to their patients' male partners, and they often respond negatively when asked if this is possible. It is undeniable—and undenied—that yeast infections in women are common. Medical experts tell us that 75% of women will experience a vaginal yeast infection in her lifetime and 40% suffer from recurrent vaginal yeast infections. What demands review is not female yeast infections, rather the role of the male partner in female yeast infections.

No, it does not require a male partner for yeast to begin growing in the vagina and other mucous membrane tissues. Antibiotics can initiate yeast overgrowth. However, the question that so many women ask their gynecologists is a logical one; what does my partner have to do with this? Many women with chronic vaginal yeast infections eventually figure out by deduction that a loving relationship with their male partners seems to precipitate the yeast infections. Whether or not a woman can get a vaginal yeast infection from a male may be questionable to male researchers, but I'll bet it is not to female researchers!

Why Do Gynecologists Not See the Connection?

There are a number of studies that show the jury is out as to whether or not males are responsible for passing yeast infections to women, and your doctor may have seen these studies. I respectfully have to question such studies for a simple, logical reason; sometimes they take place in test tubes outside of the body. We call these studies *in vitro* studies. One of these studies relied on men doing at-home swabs of their urine, feces, semen and tongue. [1] I am a man, and I have to chuckle as I ponder any man doing these tests properly himself. Lab test results are only as accurate as the preparation of the specimen being examined!

Whereas all of the female participants had to subject themselves to full OB-GYN exams to retrieve samples of their tissues, male participant simply did these tests at home and sent their samples to a laboratory where they were analyzed for the yeast responsible for most vaginal yeast infections, *Candida albicans*. What do these results have to do with skin-to-skin contact? Both female and male tissues were tested independently, and in a laboratory. How they ever arrived at their conclusion still has me shaking my head in wonder, but they did published that men are not involved in passing yeast to female partners. There is, of course, no comparison between this kind of study and what is actually happening when women and their male partner engage in skin-to-skin contact. Better studies can and must be done.

Also, consider what is missing in this study. The male skin, including that on his penis, was not tested at all! I am no genius, but I am thinking that is pretty important if we are to conclude that males do not contribute to female vaginal yeast infections. How in the world does simple logic get overlooked in medical studies? Regardless, it is important to be aware that physicians do not believe that male skin can harbor yeast or fungi.

Clinically, I believe that many doctors observe the effect (symptom) and believe it is the cause. Yes, vaginal yeast infections involved yeast. But the question many women ask is, "Why does my yeast infection come back with a vengeance each time intimacy is enjoyed if my male partner isn't somehow contributing to it?"

The answer doctors always seem to give is, *"We do not know, but take this medication."*

When you treat a symptom as if it were the cause, you will never know or treat the cause. This simple sentence might explain why the pharmaceutical industry is thriving.

There are many well known species of fungal organisms that can survive on the skin such as ringworm, jock itch, other forms of dermatitis and nail fungus. But, while the fungal disease ringworm is known to be contagious with skin to skin contact, we continue to deny that other fungi that live in more intimate areas are also spread by skin to skin contact. This makes no sense.

Getting past the Gate Keeper

As you read through this chapter, the one most important point that I hope you remember is this: Symptom and disease-causing fungi can find their way into any human tissue except the teeth. Our immune systems are the gatekeepers for anything unknown or foreign entering our body. A process called immuno-recognition enables our blood cells to immediately identify and recognize a return visitor, whereas another process called immuno-memory identifies and locks in familiar cells that were at one time foreign to our cells, rendering them safe and pre-approved for reentry. If bad cells get pre-approved initially, they likely will not be denied entry in the future, and this is where symptoms may begin.

These immune processes play an important role in sexual intimacy. The first time you have sex with someone, the immune system responds to the cells from your partner as if they were foreign invaders. It sends white blood cells to check them out and make sure they are not harmful. When they prove to be harmless, your immune system recognizes your partner's cells in future encounters and remembers how to respond to them. They get a pass similar to a TSA pre-check that lets you pass through security more quickly in the airport.

Now, let's say there is a "bad apple" in his cells. Perhaps it is a disease-causing fungus. Your immune system responds by identifying that "one in a million" cell and remembering it. Maybe that partner is never seen again, but his bad-guy fungal cell may have long-term effects on your health. One encounter like this is rarely noteworthy. But the more partners you have, the more bad guys might gain access to your body as your immune system literally falls down on the job by identifying and memorizing them. 20 bad fungal cells, all having been identified, might begin to compromise your immune system. When you have one partner, your immune system will eventually separate the bad guys from the good guys, especially if you help it with a diet that discourages fungal proliferation and a lifestyle that enhances your immunity rather than compromises it. All of this is to say that monogamy works for a reason. It helps protect you and your partner from fungi and other disease-causing germs.

How Does a Yeast Infection Get Passed Back and Forth?

Fungal organisms that thrive on the skin, hair and nails are known as dermatophytes, and they can be disease-causing (pathogenic). *Tinea cruris*, or jock itch, is a skin fungal infection that usually grows within the skin of the groin or genitals of males. A medical study in 2002 proved that jock itch and the lesions of this condition could be passed from men to women. Although the parameters of this study involved prostitutes who averaged 50 sexual partners each month, the fact remained that jock itch could be actively spread to some of the females. [2]

We also know that there are fungi on our hands, in our mouths and on every other part of our skin. Therefore, it makes sense that during sexual contact, from foreplay to intercourse, each partner is exposed to whatever organisms are living on the other partner's skin. This creates a situation by which opportunistic fungi can spread themselves by transferring between partners, even in a monogamous relationship, but less so because of immuno-memory.

Sexual contact provides multiple ways for you to become infected with any number of organisms, including these fungal organisms. Any contact with skin may provide the opportunity for fungal dermatophytes to transfer between partners. The act of sexual intercourse provides opportunities for any organism that is present on your partner to be introduced to the vaginal tract, and from there, proliferate. Recall that fungi seek modes of transportation and are thrilled when Bob finds transportation for his fungus on (or in) Sue!

Because so little is known about sexually transmitted fungal diseases, we tend to focus only on the belief that women can become infected by men, but the reverse is also true. Recall in the last chapter we pointed out that the most common prostate fungal condition, (fungal prostatitis), is caused by the yeast *Candida albicans*. This is the same fungus that causes vaginal yeast infections. During sexual intercourse, the urine tube of the male can be infected with *Candida* yeast from the female, and just a short distance up the male urine tube is the prostate gland. It can and does become infected with that yeast too.

Do you recall the ridicule that Michael Douglas received when he blamed his throat cancer on oral sex with his spouse? Now there is mounting evidence that he was right. One prominent infectious disease specialist recently stated that mouth and throat cancers were once thought to be smokers' or drinkers' diseases, but more and more, doctors are convinced that human papilloma virus (HPV) can cause these cancers. [3] If a woman has HPV, there is an increased risk of her passing this cancer-causing organism to a partner during oral sex. Most physicians now know this about viruses, but the role of fungus in spreading cancer is, unfortunately, unknown to them. It stands to reason that if viruses can be passed in this manner, fungi can be as well.

One study done in 2007 and published in the New England Journal of Medicine stated that oral sex did indeed increase the risk of oral cancers. Patients who had a lifetime number of six or more oral sex partners were 3.4 times more likely to have oropharyngeal (mouth and throat) cancer. They did not equate this increased risk to fungus, however, stating that HPV was the culprit. [4] While about 7% of the population carries oral HPV, about 50% of people have oral yeast. [5, 6] As some of you reading this know, I believe and have documented that cancer is being over-diagnosed, because fungal growths can mimic cancer. One day I hope to delve further into my studies of viral infections, because they too might mimic fungal infections. In the case of oral sex giving rise to oral cancers, just based on sheer numbers, it appears to me that oral yeast infections, not just oral viral infections, may be the culprit.

In my opinion, because antiviral vaccines and medications are flooding the market currently, much attention and money is dedicated to controlling viruses. In order to sell their wares, drug companies must flex their media muscles to make us aware of how much their wares are needed. They are selling controversial HPV vaccines in record numbers, thereby overshadowing the importance of other organisms that do not respond to vaccines, like fungus.

Fortunately, studies do exist that lead us all to believe that fungus does sexually transmit. Oral sex is known to provide the opportunity for fungal organisms and *Candida* to be spread between partners. A study published in 1996 concluded that, "Receptive oral sex has been implicated as a risk factor for vulvovaginal candidiasis..." The study went on to note that, "Oral sex may provide a route for transmission of yeast, as one-third to one-half of adults carry yeast in their oral cavity." [7] Womenshealth.gov reports that oral sex with men or with women can also spread STIs, including, rarely, HIV. HIV can potentially be passed through a mucous membrane (such as the mouth) by vaginal fluids or blood, especially if the membrane is torn or cut. [8]

Sexually Transmitted Diseases and Cancer

A study published on oral cancer rates associated with oral sex revealed that the greater number of partners one has, the more risk increases. The study indicated that for people with fewer than five partners the risk was relatively low, while risk increased with a greater number of partners. [9]

It is a commonly held notion that certain sexually transmitted diseases can cause cancer. Human papilloma virus is known to cause cancers in women and men. It is spread via vaginal, anal or oral sex. While it is thought that the virus will likely not cause any symptoms for most people, it is known to play a role in the incidence of cancer for some. [10]

Some years back, then-governor of Texas, Rick Perry, passed into law that all young girls under a certain age in Texas would receive a mandatory human papilloma virus (HPV) vaccine. This polarizing decision spurred quite a bit of rhetoric on both sides of the debate, but while some believed drug company lobbyists had their way with Governor Perry, he claimed his decision was motivated by the fact that the HPV vaccine would reduce the risk of girls developing cervical cancer caused by HPV. Regardless, the idea that an organism such as a virus can cause cancer raises very valid questions about cancer and whether other organisms may play a role in its incidence as well.

Fungal Infections of the Genitourinary Tract and UTIs

The fact that fungus can infect the genitourinary tract—the pathways out of the body that our reproductive and urinary systems share—

comes as no surprise to any woman who has had a yeast infection. To this end, women are typically prescribed a one-time pill or a number of different creams to treat the infection. This is largely the extent to which fungus is implicated and treated in the genitourinary tract of women, at least in most doctors' offices.

Unfortunately for most, if not all women with chronic yeast vaginitis, this quick treatment approach will never work, and they will continue to suffer throughout their lives. Recall the 1977 study implicating gut yeast as a major factor controlling vaginal yeast. This was reported 40+ years ago, yet gynecologists still do not know this information. Otherwise, every recurrent yeast infection would involve gynecologists teaching their patients of the gut-fungal cause, while instructing that the safe gut anti-fungal drug Nystatin along with diet and probiotic treatments would have to be carefully adhered to in order to cure their gut and vaginal yeast infections. You will not learn this in your average doctor's office, but more and more, this information is getting out.

No talk of genitourinary yeast is complete without discussing urinary tract infections (UTI) or cystitis. Whereas doctors routinely treat cystitis with antibiotics (because it is purportedly caused by bacteria), cystitis can also be caused by fungi. Again, this information is rarely known in medical offices, but it is well documented. The medical journal *Urology* documented four individual female cases of fungal cystitis. [11] I know that four cases does not lead to the definitive conclusion that cystitis is a fungal disease, but it presents a great start at understanding the role of fungus in cystitis by demonstrating that fungus can, in fact, cause cystitis.

Women with cystitis suffer horribly from urinary urgency and frequency. There is also the presence of white blood cells in the urine, indicating an infection (but not necessarily a bacterial infection), as well as blood in their urine. For the four fortunate women in the study, one can only imagine how many antibiotics had failed them before biopsies finally helped diagnose the cause of their misery; it was not bacteria, but fungus! Yet biopsies are not routinely done, so most all women are assumed to have bacterial cystitis and given antibiotics. This is tragic, but random antibiotic prescribing is not limited to UTIs.

Your Partner's Role in Cystitis

What causes cystitis? Chronic cystitis used to be called *honeymoon cystitis*. This, of course, conjures up the image of a male role in this painful condition, as well it should. As you now know, men's skin (any or all of it) can grow potentially harmful fungi called dermatophytes. They can also have other yeasts growing on their skin. These tiny fungi adhere to the skin, including the skin on the penis. The *International Journal of Dermatology* studied 261 young men aged 11 to 30 years who suffered from jock itch (*Tinea cruris*). Of the 261, about one in five (20%) had this fungus on their penises as well as their crotches. This was an Indian study, and the authors felt that the men's underwear, called langota, was partially responsible for the infections, because its tight fit favored fungal growth. [12] After reviewing photos of langota underwear online, I am hard-pressed to favor American briefs as being less conducive to fungal growth than langotas!

The problem is rarely the underwear but the lack of carefully drying the skin before slipping the underwear on. I worked for a prominent dermatologist in Dallas for several years and cannot tell you how many men with chronic jock itch I counseled. I taught them to fully and carefully blow-dry the genitalia and the crotch area after bathing each day, and then switch to boxer type underwear, enabling the skin to breath. That approach really worked for these men. But, most importantly, by lowering their skin fungus load, they have also lowered their ability to pass these skin fungi along to their spouses as they maintained their loving relationships. Everyone but the fungi benefited!

When I first began working with various doctors in clinical nutritional settings, it was particularly interesting to me how commonly the alcohol-consuming male (who is consuming yeast and mycotoxins in the alcohol) seemed to pass toxic yeast spores from his gut to his skin, thereby inflaming sensitive tissues in the female when skin to skin contact was made. This was just my hypothesis, mind you. I still feel that men and women who consume alcohol are more vulnerable to fungal growth anywhere in their bodies. Condoms, I would teach, protect both partners in cases where alcohol consumption might be considered an important contributing factor. I found that a few supplements and a changed lifestyle would alleviate many problems that yeast was provoking.

Sex Lubricants, Feminine Hygiene and Yeast Problems

Painful intercourse may have more to do with fungal organisms than was ever previously thought, and both partners need to know this. We now know that yeast infections of the vaginal tract are not uncommon, and for many women they are a chronic condition. Many causes can be implicated from diet, high blood sugar and high estrogen levels, to a recent round of antibiotics. [13]

One less commonly implicated exacerbation of yeast infections is sexual lubricants and feminine hygiene products. Most of these products are typically made with a base of glycerin, silicone or essential oils. As it turns out, glycerin is an excellent platform for growing *Candida* yeast. Subsequently, using glycerin-based lubricants may play a role in the incidence and frequency of *Candida* infections in the vagina. Most douche products contain the same bases, and they are of course wet, which provides an environment fungi love.

Women who use lubricants and feminine hygiene products may be inadvertently harboring fungi. These organisms not only contribute to their own yeast infections, but these women may also be passing these infections to their husbands through sexual contact.

Fungus and HIV

Human immunodeficiency virus, or HIV, is a terrible disease that has claimed the lives of many people. It is transferred via contact with sexual fluid and blood. Once the virus progresses into AIDS, sufferers of the disease are left with a completely compromised immune system. Without immuno-memory and immuno-recognition, they unfortunately become vulnerable to any germ that comes their way, and the immune system's gates, once guarded, are now wide open.

It is interesting to note that Pfizer's blockbuster drug, Diflucan, which went on sale in the 1980s, was initially aimed at treating AIDS. In 1996, the Center For Disease Control (CDC) posted this fact on their website, cdc.gov, "Fungal diseases are increasing among patients infected with human immunodeficiency virus (HIV) type 1. Infections due to *Candida* and *Cryptococcus* are the most common." [14]

Pfizer's new drug, Diflucan, fit the bill perfectly, as it treated both of these fungal infections with relative safety. But the fact that an anti-fungal drug successfully treated thousands of AIDS patients really got me thinking; are we mistaking a fungal infection for a viral infection? Surely medical science would scoff at such an idea, but it does raise an interesting question.

A few years later, Pfizer was granted an additional use for Diflucan. It became known in medical clinics as the one-pill vaginal yeast cure. How does a pill that only kills fungus become a best selling AIDS drug if a virus causes AIDS? Diflucan does not kill viruses. That leaves the question as to whether AIDS might be more fungal in nature than viral. Again, it is important that you know that current medical science completely disagrees with some of my hypotheses.

The answer may lie in questioning our diagnostic abilities more than the germ responsible. Once again, sometimes doctors see the effect of the disease and mistake it for the cause. Giving it a name solidifies this mistake. A lump, for example, is called cancer. High blood sugar is called diabetes. Disregarding what caused the lump or the high blood sugar has made the pharmaceutical industry wealthy, but have you and I really benefitted other than living a life relegated to buying their wares?

Many HIV and AIDS patients are at risk for developing fungal infections, and as many as 50% can prove to be fatal, but diagnosticians see those as secondary infections. [15] The primary infection, they learn, is viral. At the beginning of this book, however, we noted that fungi impede human immune systems. With a compromised immune system and no way to fend off opportunistic fungi, fungal infections are free to proliferate throughout the body.

The fungus link to HIV doesn't stop there. There is evidence to support that vaginal yeast increases the likelihood of contracting HIV. In a study published in 2003, Robin Hester and Dr. Stephen Kennedy wrote, "Women who seroconverted (blood tested) from HIV-negative status during baseline to HIV-positive status at follow-up were significantly more likely to have vaginal *Candida* infections than were the correspondingly matched seronegative control women." [16] In plain English, this is saying that women whose blood tested HIV-positive were much more likely to have yeast infections than those whose blood tested HIV-negative.

A few years ago, I posted a blog review of an amazing science article. I coined the name, *HIF*, referring to *Human Immuno Fungus*. My blog was a review of a study on AIDS, HIV and mycotoxins in African patients which stated, "Leading theories suggest that the fungal toxin may suppress the immune system by reducing the production of certain immune cells or the proteins that activate them. The toxin also may increase the expression of genes that result in more copies of the virus, but more study is needed to confirm the mechanisms." [17]

Notice what is not mentioned. Perhaps—just perhaps—fungus was at the root of the infections and not a secondary bystander.

AIDS stands for acquired immunodeficiency syndrome. HIV stands for human immunodeficiency virus. They are related conditions. The African diet is rich in corn and peanuts. Corn and peanuts are often infected with *Aspergillus* mold. *Aspergillus* mold makes aflatoxin, a poisonous mycotoxin. In the study, two tubes of blood were drawn from 314 African AIDS patients. One tube from each patient is tested for HIV. The other tube is tested for mold (aflatoxin). Positive HIV tests are then tested for what is known as a "viral load," which varies depending upon how much HIV is in the blood.

The higher the mold count was in the blood, the higher the HIV viral load was. Does this not lend credibility of, at very least, fungal involvement in AIDS? Is the HIV test a mold test or a viral test? Does HIV exist when fungus is the cause? Should HIV be immediately renamed *HIF*?

Again, my hypotheticals are here merely to keep your brain thinking. Decades from now, when I'm gone, these included hypothesis might just account for rapid book sales as they are proven correct...or not.

Putting Our Knowledge to Work

We now have a pretty good understanding of what fungus is, what it does and how it gets into your body. For the rest of the book, we will focus on specific types of health challenges that are caused or made worse by fungus. The solutions will be a recurring theme, and that is okay. I formulated the Kaufmann Lifestyle and the Kaufmann Diet specifically to address all fungal infections since they are so common, given our lifestyle habits and our SAD way of eating.

You may want to read each chapter in succession, but you are free to skip to the chapters most pertinent to your needs. You can come back to them when you are done, or you can pass the book on to someone who does have them. Better yet, you can keep your copy for reference and order one for your friends or loved ones.

Let the healing begin!

References:
(1) University Of Michigan Health System. "Men Do Not Cause Yeast Infections In Women, Study Finds." *ScienceDaily*, 19 December 2003)
(2) Otero, L, et al. "Tinea Cruris in Female Prostitutes." *Mycopathologia*, vol. 153, no. 1, 2002, pp. 29–31.
(3) Catharine Paddock, PhD, "Oral Sex Increases Throat Cancer Risk Scientists Say", accessed July 7, 2016, http://www.medicalnewstoday.com/articles/70495.php.
(4) Dsouza, Gypsyamber, et al. "Case–Control Study of Human Papillomavirus and Oropharyngeal Cancer." *New England Journal of Medicine*, vol. 356, no. 19, Oct. 2007, pp. 1944–1956., doi:10.1056/nejmoa065497.
(5) "HPV and Oropharyngeal Cancer–Fact Sheet", accessed July 7, 2016, http://www.cdc.gov/std/hpv/stdfact-hpvandoropharyngealcancer.htm.
(6) "Oral thrush (fungal infection in the mouth)", accessed July 7, 2016, http://www.netdoctor.co.uk/diseases/facts/oralthrush.htm.
(7) Geiger, Ann M., and Foxman Betsy. "Risk Factors for Vulvovaginal Candidiasis: A Case-Control Study among University Students." Epidemiology 7, no. 2 (1996): 182-87. http://www.jstor.org/stable/3703033.

(8) "Lesbian and bisexual health fact sheet", accessed July 7, 2016, http://women-shealth.gov/publications/our-publications/fact-sheet/lesbian-bisexual-health.html.

(9) Li, Sheng, et al. "Oral Sex and Risk of Oral Cancer: a Meta-Analysis of Observational Studies." *Journal of Evidence-Based Medicine*, vol. 8, no. 3, 2015, pp. 126–133., doi:10.1111/jebm.12159.

(10) "Genital HPV Infection–Fact Sheet", accessed July 7, 2016, http://www.cdc.gov/std/hpv/stdfact-hpv.htm.

(11) TJ Rohner, Jr, RM Tuliszewski, "Fungal cystitis: awareness, diagnosis and treatment," *The Journal of Urology*, 1980, 124(1):142-4, accessed July 7, 2016, http://www.ncbi.nlm.nih.gov/pubmed/7411704.

(12) SS Pandey, S Chandra, PK Guha, P Kaur, G Singh, "Dermatophyte infection of the penis. Association with a particular undergarment.", *International Journal of Dermatology*, 1981, 20(2):112-4, accessed July 7, 2016, http://www.ncbi.nlm.nih.gov/pubmed/7216591.

(13) "Vaginal Yeast Infections–Cause", accessed July 7, 2016, http://www.webmd.com/women/tc/vaginal-yeast-infections-cause.

(14) Neil M. Ampel, "Emerging Disease Issues and Fungal Pathogens Associated with HIV Infection", accessed July 7, 2016, http://wwwnc.cdc.gov/eid/article/2/2/96-0205_article.

(15) Darius Armstrong-James, Graeme Meintjes, Gordon D. Brown, "A neglected epidemic: fungal infections in HIV/AIDS", *Trends in Microbiology*, March 2014, Vol.22(3):120–127, doi:10.1016/j.tim.2014.01.001, http://www.sciencedirect.com/science/article/pii/S0966842X1400002X.

(16) RA Hester and SB Kennedy, "Candida infection as a risk factor for HIV transmission", *Journal of Women's Health*, June 2003, Vol12(5):487-94, doi:10.1089/154099903766651612, https://www.ncbi.nlm.nih.gov/pubmed/12869296.

(17) University of Alabama at Birmingham. "Is a common food fungus worsening the AIDS epidemic?." *ScienceDaily*, accessed July 7, 2016, http://www.sciencedaily.com/releases/2013/07/130723095207.htm.

CHAPTER 4

I Don't Have a Fungal Problem! I Have an Autoimmune Disorder!

People who suffer from autoimmune disorders can tell you what a frustrating and disheartening ordeal it is to live through. For most other conditions, you go to the doctor, they tell you what is wrong with you, and you go home with a treatment plan. Not so with autoimmune disorders. The path to diagnosis is long and fraught with the 3 Ds: drugs, disbelief and depression.

I understand this, but when doctors do not know the answer to your health problem immediately, their first instinct is to help you get better by trying various approaches. If none of them work, they order tests, tests and more tests. Many doctors admit that they are over testing their patients, but I do understand this. They are honestly trying to find the cause of whatever is making you sick, and certain tests might indicate the cause. Of course, the test results usually all come back saying you are fine, but you know you are not. This is frustrating to say the least.

Since they are doctors, this is where the going gets tough for you. They will tell you the test results and the results of their examinations which reveal that they can't find anything wrong with you. But being good people and really wanting to help, they continue to search for answers. Now you begin to wonder if this illness isn't all in your head! You question your own judgment of the one thing you know better than anyone else—your own body. This gets depressing as you work so hard to convince yourself that these symptoms are not really there when, in fact, not only are they there, but they are getting worse.

You buck up the courage yet again to tell either this same doctor or a succession of doctors that you know it does not make sense, but you are sick—very sick! When your determination finally outlasts their disbelief, they run more tests, prescribe more drugs and your misery continues.

Finally, after several years of this, one doctor tells you the words that make no sense in any true biological fashion: "*Your body is attacking itself.*" When you first hear this, you have one of two reactions. Either you ask, "Why in the world would my body attack itself?" Or, you experience momentary relief as you accept what finally sounds like an explanation.

But is it really? Does it not raise more questions? Does anyone know why the body would attack itself or even if the body is capable of actually attacking itself?

If you were not depressed when the tests came back negative, or if you were not depressed when they told you it is probably nothing, or if you were not depressed when you were handed antidepressants, there is now a very real chance that you will be depressed because you've just learned that this mysterious, horrible sickness is your own fault. You must have been sleeping when your body bought the boxing gloves and starting fighting itself! Most people with autoimmune disorders take long-term or permanent pharmaceutical treatments, and many end up trading the discomfort of their disorder for the discomfort of drug side effects. For many, depression is the least of their worries as the illness worsens. Your doctor kindly offers you antidepressants.

Doctors and Medical Researchers Are Very Bright People

As you have already learned, when your body detects any sort of foreign invader, it launches an immune response. *Antigen* is the catchall term for anything capable of causing an immune response. Antigens include bacteria, cancer cells, toxins, viruses, fungi, cat dander, wheat and anything else your body must deal with. In a normal, healthy body, the immune system can distinguish between cells that belong there and cells that do not. In the case of autoimmune disease, however, the immune system does not distinguish between foreign antigens and normal bodily tissue. Subsequently, doctors believe that healthy tissues are attacked by…other healthy tissues. While there are differences between the specific kinds of autoimmune diseases, this, they learn, is generally how autoimmune diseases work. These are "mistakes" of the immune system. You learn that your immune system isn't working correctly.

Autoimmune diseases (AD) are rather unique among the diseases discussed in this book in that medical researchers have gone below the surface to try to figure them out. When researchers peer down the eyepiece of a microscope at a culture of cells from a person with telltale symptoms of an autoimmune disorder, what they see looks for all the world like healthy cells are attacking each other. The cells doing the attacking are the standard white blood cells in all their varieties. That is no surprise. What is odd is that the cells being attacked look like healthy cells from healthy tissues. There is no explanation for why this is happening, or so they are taught. For many years they have had no good reason to think otherwise. But maybe there is a better explanation for your misery.

If you think fungi are tiny, imagine how small the solids, liquids or gasses their poisonous mycotoxins are. They are absolutely invisible to the naked eye. It is difficult to diagnose what you cannot see, but you can see human cells and other tissues killing each other, so therein lies your diagnosis.

While there are over 135 identified autoimmune diseases known to scientists today according to the National Institute of Health (NIH), "The exact cause of autoimmune disorders is unknown." So while we have a general understanding of what these diseases look like, and a general idea of what symptoms each produces in patients, modern medicine is unsure of what necessarily kick starts the process that leads to any one of these diseases.

We are commonly exposed to fungus; our food, medications and air supply are filled with fungi. What if autoimmune disorders were due to invisible poisons infecting your blood and organs? You would be miserable, and doctors wouldn't know why. Isn't that exactly where you are now? Welcome to the world of autoimmune diseases.

Current Treatment

I know that everything doctors are doing for autoimmune disorders is done with the patient's best interest in mind. You are hurting, and they wholeheartedly believe that your immune system is not functioning. In essence, when an autoimmune disorder is diagnosed, the fault lies with you! I believe indirectly that may be true, since you inadvertently invited fungus to live with you. But by addressing and treating it if it is the problem, you should improve. Since doctors and research scientists believe that the tissues under attack are healthy in autoimmune disorders, they have turned almost all of their attention to your immune system. Their objective is to find ways to suppress your immune system, since that is obviously the problem, or rather, it is *apparently* the problem. The trick is to suppress the immune system enough to keep it from continuing to attack your body, but not so much that it fails to protect you from other diseases. The concept is analogous to chemotherapy; kill the cancer cells before you kill the patient. (More on cancer later!)

Reducing immunity is a problem itself, because there are simply so many functions and variables within your immune system. While treating autoimmune disorders with immune suppressing drugs, isn't the doctor making the patient more susceptible to germ infections of all kinds, including fungus? And therein lies the biggest problem—not understanding that it may be fungus that is causing this problem to begin with! When immunity is lowered opportunistic germs like fungus thrive. If it is fungus causing your autoimmune disorder, you'll continue to get worse and worse as fungi continue to increase in numbers inside you. So, like other autoimmune patients, you get sicker throughout the months and years, and no one ever figures out that the very immune-suppressing treatment you are taking has enabled the offending fungi to simply hold the immune system gates open for their poisons to walk right in. The death certificate never states "chronic mycotoxicosis" as the cause of death. Instead, the clever name chosen for the autoimmune disease is blamed for your death. In essence, according to our researchers today, you fought yourself to death. Does that make sense?

There are five major types of blood cells that make up the majority of your immune system, and there are dozens of varieties among them.

There are 4,000-11,000 of them per *microliter* (cc) in your blood. (For reference, there are 20,000 microliters in a 2-liter bottle of pop.) Immune cells help combat disease-causing species of bacteria, viruses, fungi and other toxins. To strike the balance in the middle of all those factors, you have to be able to nurture and maintain complete control over all of them. It makes herding cats seem like a breeze!

Autoimmune Diseases and Women

Given that young, childbearing aged women are more vulnerable to autoimmune diseases, let's try to figure out why. Sadly, almost one half of these women are labeled as chronic complainers (in this sense, "complainer" simply means one who reports a problem), which almost makes sense given how long it takes to diagnose an autoimmune disease. According to the American Autoimmune Related Disease Association, Inc (AARDA), *it takes most women about 4.6 years and about 5 different doctors before they are finally accurately diagnosed with autoimmune disorders.*

Did I say accurately? Given the number of doctors involved and the length of time needed to try to diagnose autoimmune disorders, by this time your disease is fairly advanced, and you are deservedly upset. Your strange symptoms now have a name, but how that name gets you better is yet another subject. Why did this happen to you?

No one knows why women are more vulnerable to autoimmune disorders, and since no one knows, I'd like to take a shot at why. A 2001 Center for Disease Control (CDC) study entitled, *New Study Profiles Women's Use of Health Care*, published that women go to doctors—lots of doctors. The average woman goes to 4.6 doctors annually. This means that during their childbearing years (from 20 to 35 years of age), women will have, on average, 69 doctor office visits! [1] Believe me when I tell you, doctors are taught to diagnose, and they are very good at it. If, during just one of those 69 visits, a woman complains of a chronic rash or a spell of dizziness, lab tests will be recommended… and the cycle of begins. That's just my take, but there is reasoning behind my take. Consider this: We are told that from time to time, we all make cancer cells in our bodies. The odds of a doctor seeing those cancer cells increases when we go to them! I'm a male who got the flu in 2017 and went to a local care facility for an antibiotic. In 2006, I was knocked off my bicycle by a truck and ended up in an emergency room, where I denied all treatments, including surgery for a dislocated shoulder and powerful pain medications. Prior to those two events, my last physical examination was my exit physical from the U.S. Navy in 1972. That was 47 years ago! Can you imagine how many cancer cells I've made during those 46 years that were not detected by a doctor? And that is exactly my point.

Woman are taught by their mothers to go to doctors. Knowing this, clever medical advertising began to surface long ago. Random doctor visits became known as *"annuals."* Remember that? Marketing changed the direction of medical screenings. Then it became, "Women, make certain you get your *annual* pap smear and mammogram." No one seemed to question this approach, and doctors' offices and pharmacies were constantly filled—and thrilled. The plan was working perfectly. They tried it with men, too, but to no one's surprise, male annual rectal exams just didn't seem to be catching on. So, a bad blood test called the PSA was invented and (combined with fear tactics) was very successfully marketed, I believe to the detriment of both men and mankind.

Fortunately, this is all changing. In the past decade, the word *"annual,"* within a physical examination context, has been questioned even by medical authorities. A 2013 report on the medical website, Medscape.com, reads: *"Unnecessary Pap Tests In Millions Of US Woman."* The report noted, "In their report on cervical cancer screening released yesterday, the Centers for Disease Control and Prevention (CDC) startlingly estimated that 22 million women in the United States may have undergone such screening unnecessarily, because they had already had hysterectomies."

This clandestine cheating should shock every American, but we simply went on with our lives, trusting that all was well within the halls of science. Newer screening guidelines are now eliminating the word "annual" in female pap testing in healthy women.

Mammography is yet another story. In 2014, after following mammography reports on 90,000 women ages 40-59 for 25 years, the prestigious British Medical Journal concluded, "Annual mammography in women aged 40-59 does not reduce mortality from breast cancer beyond that of physical examination or usual care when adjuvant therapy from breast cancer is freely available. Overall, 22% of screen(ings) detected invasive breast cancers were over-diagnosed." In other words, 22% of mammograms were *false positive readings*. [2]

Given that about 20% of mammograms have *false negative readings* [3], women are left with a "gold standard" breast cancer diagnostic test that has been used for decades, that on average is actually about 58% accurate. Did you know that? Does your doctor know this? As I previously mentioned, I wanted to present information in this book that you may be unfamiliar with for you to share with your doctor. The two of you should meet and discuss continued cancer screenings based on his/her knowledge of your health history and not based on information within this book. This is important.

The term, *over diagnosed*, from the British Medical Journal is relevant. Because women are visiting their doctors in record numbers, my concern is that many are being over diagnosed not only with breast cancer but with autoimmune disorders as well.

With such a broad scope of misery, you can imagine the amount of money that gets poured into research on a yearly basis with the intention of fighting autoimmune disease. Despite all the money and research hours spent, the exact cause of autoimmune disease is still to be officially determined. However, the lack of a known cause has not stopped the arrival of blockbuster drugs used to treat autoimmune disease symptoms, nor has it stopped drug companies from investing in new drugs and making billions of dollars by hushing symptoms a few hours at a time.

What is the cause of these autoimmune diseases? What is going on in a woman's life and in her body at childbearing age that would make her so vulnerable? I believe we deserve a better explanation than "her cells started fighting one another" as the cause of these mysterious illnesses. As you are learning, what I want to teach you in this book is a brand new explanation for age-old diseases. What was done in the past obviously did not work, or autoimmune disease would be shrinking in number of people affected rather than dramatically growing.

One of two things is going to happen. We must either continue producing mass quantities of new medication, or think differently. Now, let's look at the different types of autoimmune diseases that exist, and then I promise we will come back to thinking differently. What you will learn will amaze you.

Common Autoimmune Diseases

This is information that our doctors learn about the most common anti-immune diseases. By learning this, perhaps we can create a new way of thinking about their causes.

Rheumatoid Arthritis

Rheumatoid arthritis, or RA, is an autoimmune disease that primarily affects the joints but usually involves other organs as well. Joints are usually affected in a symmetrical pattern, and those commonly affected include fingers, hands, elbows, shoulders, knees and ankles. In cases of RA, the immune system attacks the synovium, or the lining of the membrane surrounding joints. This causes painful, swollen joints and destroys the cartilage and bones of the joints. Rheumatoid arthritis also increases the risk of heart and lung problems.

Rheumatoid arthritis is typically treated with steroids as a first line of defense, but other drugs such as disease-modifying, anti-rheumatic drugs (DMARDs) like methotrexate, or a newer class of drugs known as biologics are beginning to appear. Biologics are often paired with another DMARD for maximum effectiveness. Side effects associated with these types of drugs are not to be taken lightly. They can cause damage to the liver and increase the risk of infections.

Systemic Lupus

Lupus is a chronic, inflammatory condition that affects multiple organ systems. It can affect the joints, skin, brain, blood cells, heart and lungs. Since no two cases of lupus are necessarily the same, it can be difficult to diagnose, but the most telling symptom of someone with lupus is a butterfly–like rash spreading across the face. Lupus is the Latin word for bunny, and the rash looks a bit like a bunny mask, hence the name.

Lupus attacks multiple organ systems and can damage to the kidneys, brain, central nervous system, lungs, heart, blood and blood vessels. Kidney failure is among the leading cause of death for lupus patients. Treating lupus, like treatment for other autoimmune diseases, may involve a combination of drugs including anti-malarial drugs, cortico-steroids and immune-suppressing drugs such as methotrexate.

It is thought that lupus is caused by a combination of genetics and en-vironmental factors. Infections can trigger lupus or instigate a relapse. Doctors will admit, however, the cause generally remains unknown.

Multiple Sclerosis (MS)

Multiple Sclerosis, doctors learn, is a disease in which the immune system damages the myelin sheath surrounding nerves. Over time, this can cause nerve damage. Many patients will lose the ability to walk independently. Symptoms include numbness or weakness in one or more limbs, prolonged double vision, partial or complete vision loss, tingling or pain in parts of the body, electric shock sensations with certain neck movements, tremors, slurred speech, dizziness or problems with bowel or bladder.

By now you can probably guess that MS is treated with a variety of immunosuppressant drugs. The exact cause remains unknown, but like other autoimmune diseases, scientists believe genetic and envi-ronmental factors are to blame.

Fibromylagia

Fibromyalgia is a condition characterized by fatigue, cognitive problems or "brain fog" and widespread, dull pain. People with fibro-myalgia tend to experience fatigue even after long periods of sleep. The fatigue and pain associated with fibromyalgia can interfere with the work and personal life of those who suffer from the condition. Fibromyalgia can be notoriously difficult to diagnose—it can take as long as 3-5 years to get a diagnosis for some patients.

It is thought that infections and genetics might play a role, but the exact cause of fibromyalgia remains unknown.

During the past 25 years, we have seen an explosion of fibromyalgia diagnoses. I do not recall being able to pronounce it nor anyone having it in 1985, but over 5 million Americans have it today, almost 90% being female. According to womenshealth.gov, the causes of fibromyalgia are not known. (*For these and other reasons, the topic of fibromyalgia deserves, and will get, its own chapter in this book.*)

Thyroid Disease

The thyroid gland is a gland in the neck which produces thyroid hormones that help regulate most metabolic functions in the body. Thyroid diseases fall into two categories: hyperthyroid disease and hypothyroid disease.

In the case of hyperthyroid disease (Graves' Disease), the thyroid produces too much thyroid hormone. Symptoms include irritability, anxiety, heart palpitations, tremors, heat and light sensitivity, weight loss, libido changes, menstrual changes and bulging eyes. Graves' Disease can lead to heart problems and cause problems with pregnancy. It is often treated with radioactive iodine, anti-thyroid drugs or surgery.

In the case of hypothyroid disease (Hashimoto's Disease), the thyroid produces too little thyroid hormone. Symptoms include weight gain, fatigue, slowed heart rate, irregular periods, difficulty getting pregnant, depression, inability to get warm and joint/muscle pain. Hashimoto's is treated with hormone replacements. It is thought that infections and genetics play a role in its incidence. How close they are I believe!

Thinking Differently

While we have plenty of treatments to aid in mitigating the ravages of these autoimmune diseases, there is no cure available for any one of the 135 of them. Blaming our genes for everything that ails us is no longer fashionable even in medical circles. There is one important aspect of autoimmunity that science has yet to acknowledge as playing a role in their development. It is why I disagree with the concept of autoimmunity, altogether.

I don't believe that the human body is attacking itself. Nowhere in nature does any healthy organism with the ability to defend itself turn and attack itself. When the underlying cause of a disease or symptoms is unknown or poorly understood, it is time to at least consider a pathogen or poison that is both invisible and not well understood among the medical establishment—especially one that, when it has been studied, has been known to affect people at the molecular level and cause much ill health. We know with certainty that human liver cancer has been caused by a fungal mycotoxin. Why not autoimmune disease?

If you look back at the suspected causes of all the major autoimmune diseases, they all mention environmental factors. Researchers are definitely on the right track. Remember that fungi, their spores and their mycotoxins, like autoimmune diseases, are everywhere. This means they are contaminants of the environment that we inhabit. We have also established repeatedly that fungi and mycotoxins contaminate our food supply—this is well documented. This fact has even begun piquing the interest of medical researchers.

For many readers, different thinking calls for an abundance of caution. Just because we are exposed to these pathogens and their poisons does not necessarily mean that we should automatically claim them as the cause of autoimmune disease. We need more evidence, and there is plenty.

Fungi are constantly working to break down the environment they inhabit, and the mycotoxins they produce work towards this end. Organ systems that have been ravaged by autoimmune disease show the effects of literally being severely damaged and broken down. So, that is our first clue that fungi and their mycotoxins could be to blame!

Recent research into the sub-cellular behavior of mycotoxins has revealed something promising in terms of understanding autoimmune disease, yet horribly disturbing in terms of what is really going on. Certain mycotoxins have shown an ability to penetrate cell walls without destroying them. They move in, kill the part of the cell responsible for reproduction, and take its place. They can then make copies of cells just like them. So it is almost like a carjacking, where the thief can then replicate the car *and* the driver. When past researchers have looked at cell cultures of people with autoimmune disease, they have only seen the car. They did not know to look at the driver.

This is why I have speculated for years that our immune systems could be confusing healthy tissue for something that is actually infecting the tissue, such as a deep-seated fungal infection. We know that fungi can infect nearly every tissue in the human body. We know, too, that most fungal mycotoxins inhibit normal immune system function. Healthy human cells and fungal cells have DNA within their nuclei. Might DNA from healthy human cells merge with fungal DNA? Such a merger would create a hybrid structure that our brightest and best researchers would have never seen and therefore would be unable to recognize or diagnose. The entire time, your blood cells would appear to be being attacked. As hybrid cells metastasized, the only thing a doctor could do would be to treat the symptoms without regard to a cause, which he could not see.

I know that this sounds a bit like science fiction, but many viruses—the Epstein-Barr virus, papilloma viruses, and hepatitis B and C viruses—promote human cancers by integrating their DNA into human cells. [4] Consider also that a 1996 medical textbook published that fungi were capable of altering human immune systems in favor of its own survival! [5] These are tricky germs that will stop at nothing to gain access to a warm environment that is filled with food.

But perhaps one of the most interesting facts about autoimmune disorders is that physicians prescribe antibiotics to the patients with them. Are there any autoimmune disease patients that have not had rounds of antibiotics hoping to fix the problem? In 2014, a research paper headline surfaced that spoke of antibiotics and their use on patients with autoimmune disorders: "Antibiotics have been applied for the treatment of autoimmune diseases for over five decades, based on the premise that infections play a role in the initiation and propagation of these entities." [6]

They are 50% correct in believing that germs cause autoimmune disorders, but that makes them 50% wrong, and they might unknowingly be placing autoimmune patients at risk when prescribing antibiotics. While I applaud these and many other scientists for having open minds regarding a possible infectious germ as the cause of autoimmune disorders, I am shocked that anyone would pour gasoline (antibiotics, AKA, fungal mycotoxins) on a fire (autoimmune disorder of unknown cause) in hopes of putting it out. Yet pour they have done. I remain convinced today that antibiotics assure the worsening and chronicity of fungal-caused, acute disorders. I have helped so many people with autoimmune disorders by safely addressing a possible fungal role to their autoimmune disorder that I am certain many, if not most, of these disorders have a fungal base.

My hypothesis as to why we are seeing an explosion of young, child-bearing age women being diagnosed with autoimmune disorders has already been discussed in previous chapters of this book. Young women are visiting doctors in record numbers. For this reason and others, so many have been prescribed antibiotics, even as children. They are now grown and drinking alcohol, eating fungal-promoting diets, perhaps living in mold-infested environments and having loving sexual relationship with their spouses. As you have learned, any one of these alone could feasibly begin a chain reaction of events that might cause someone to have strange symptoms. Strange symptoms, however, do not a disease make. Scientists who study fungal disorders teach us that by combining multiple mycotoxins, the probability that illness would be provoked grows tremendously. What have you to lose by asking your doctor for a short course of anti-fungal medications and adhering to the Kaufmann Lifestyle for a month or two if you suffer from an autoimmune disorder?

A Simple Test

What you will likely hear from your rheumatologist or internist is that autoimmune diseases are incurable. Their best answers seem to doom you to a lifetime of doctor visits, prescription medication and coping with your disease. The idea that fungi or mycotoxins could influence autoimmune disease, however, is not likely something you will hear for a few decades. Regardless, a simple experimental test might reveal if fungus may be influencing your autoimmune disease. If after 30-60 days on the strictest form of the Kaufmann Diet and Lifestyle you feel much better, you may have isolated the elusive "environmental factor" implicated in autoimmune disease all along. Fungus, once inside your body, must eat to survive, and you may have erroneously been told that your diet has no impact on your disease. As I've long said, "Let them be wrong, but don't let them be dead wrong!"

Don't believe that because you feel better in 30 or 60 days you have cured your autoimmune disease. Rather, you have finally discovered from whence it came. More of the same should slowly continue to prove that hope exists. This isn't easy, but the alternative could be lifelong and worse.

References:
(1) "New Study Profiles Women's Use of Health Care." *Centers for Disease Control and Prevention*, Centers for Disease Control and Prevention, 22 Jan. 2010, www.cdc.gov/nchs/pressroom/01news/newstudy.htm.
(2) Miller, A. B., et al. "Twenty Five Year Follow-up for Breast Cancer Incidence and Mortality of the Canadian National Breast Screening Study: Randomised Screening Trial." *Bmj*, vol. 348, no. feb11 9, Nov. 2014, doi:10.1136/bmj.g366.
(3) "Limitations of Mammograms." *American Cancer Society*, www.cancer.org/cancer/breast-cancer/screening-tests-and-early-detection/mammograms/limitations-of-mammograms.html.
(4) Meurman, Jukka H. "Oral Microbiota and Cancer." *Journal of Oral Microbiology*, vol. 2, no. 1, 2010, p. 5195., doi:10.3402/jom.v2i0.5195.
(5) Kibbler, C. C., et al. *Principles and Practice of Clinical Mycology*. Wiley, 2005.
(6) Rosman, Yossi, et al. "Antibiotic Therapy in Autoimmune Disorders." *Clinical Practice*, vol. 11, no. 1, 2014, pp. 91–103., doi:10.2217/cpr.13.84.

Autoimmune Case Study and Solutions

I want to acknowledge a debt of gratitude to Dr. Lynn Jennings, MD, whose excellent newsletter regularly features case studies that demonstrate the presence of fungus in women's health conditions. These newsletters were published 7-10 years ago.

The case studies in this book are based on these newsletters unless otherwise noted. I have edited her original writing with her permission to fit our purposes, and we changed names for the sake of privacy. In every other manner, these cases are real. These are real women with real health problems that have been identified as being caused by fungi, thanks to the superb sleuth work of Dr. Jennings. You might notice in some of these that she mentions subjects we have already covered. I have left these points in for the sake of repetition, which is a good learning tool.

As you read this book and your knowledge expands, you may find yourself being able to identify health problems earlier and earlier. While this is good for your own knowledge, the studies presented in this book are for educational purposes only and should not be used as a substitute for an examination and/or treatment by a licensed health care provider.

Thyroid Problems and Fungus

For legal purposes I must always give this disclaimer: This case study is for educational purposes only. I am using it to show you how a typical patient presents and the things I consider when I make a diagnosis. The patient's name has been changed to protect her identity. I practice integrative/alternative medicine, and my recommendations for treatment are often considered outside traditional practice. It is not my intent to criticize or denounce traditional medicine. I am merely providing an alternative opinion. Most importantly, the information provided here should not be used as a substitute for an examination and treatment by a licensed health care provider.

Presenting illness:
Jennifer is a 36-year-old female who presented to the clinic for an alternative medicine consult. She had listed the following on her patient information sheet: fatigue (chronic) and sleepiness, muscle weakness, decreased sex drive, low immune system, overweight, dry skin, infertility, depression-anxiety, premenstrual syndrome (PMS), joint and muscle pain, headaches, intolerance to cold and heat, memory impairments, hair loss, high cholesterol, low vitamin D, swelling, slow digestion and dry eyes.

Medications:
Jennifer takes Clonazepam for anxiety, Tylenol with codeine for menstrual cramps and ibuprofen as needed for pain.

Allergies:
Jennifer has no known drug allergies.

Past surgical history:
Jennifer has had her wisdom teeth extracted and a cyst removed from her neck.

Social history:
Jennifer is married. She is a high school teacher. She previously smoked tobacco but has quit for over ten years. She rarely drinks alcoholic beverages. She does not exercise. Jennifer is not following any specific diet, and she does use artificial sweeteners. She has traveled outside of the United States to Europe and Mexico.

Review of systems:
In addition to her presenting illness concerns, Jennifer reports that she believes she has thyroid issues. Her father and grandmother have hypothyroidism. She reports that the hair on her legs has stopped growing. Jennifer states that she has problems with constipation. In addition to her headaches she also has a history of migraines. With regards to her PMS symptoms, Jennifer reports

that her menstrual cycle is irregular and that she has severe cramping and heavy menstrual bleeding. She states that she snores at night. Jennifer also has suffered with psoriasis. She also states that she received multiple courses of antibiotics when she was younger. She has problems with recurrent sinus infections. She reports that when she was diagnosed with low vitamin D, she was placed on an injection of 50,000 units of vitamin D per week for one month. The school where she is employed is very old. The remainder of her review of systems is unremarkable.

Physical exam:
Blood pressure: 112/76, pulse: 68, height: 5'9", weight: 231 lbs.

Jennifer has mild suborbital edema as well as thinning of her lateral eyebrows. Her tongue is pale in color, prominently scalloped and very thick. The tissues of her neck and face appear swollen.

Her skin shows mild beta carotenemia of her palms and soles. Her skin is dry. Her hands are edematous and appear "puffy". She has tenderness to palpation of the muscles of her arms. Her feet and hands are noticeably cool to the touch. Jennifer has tightness in the muscles of her neck and back.

The remainder of her physical exam was unremarkable.

Discussion:
When a patient comes into the office with a long list of symptoms, it is because traditional medicine has failed them. Many times these individuals are dismissed by their family doctors as being depressed. In Jennifer's case, the medications she takes are only designed to cover up the symptoms. They do not address the underlying cause. Fortunately, Jennifer is intelligent enough to know that she needs to take charge of her own health.

If you are familiar with Doug Kaufmann's work, then you probably have a good idea what I am going to say in this next sentence. Jennifer has chronic fungal disease.

Jennifer did not get this way overnight. She has too many symptoms. If all of this had started at once, she would not have been able to drag herself out of bed. In fact, she would still be there. As it is, she is working full time as a high school teacher. I suspect that her problems began when she was much younger. How can I say this? Jennifer self-reported that she had been on lots of antibiotics when she was younger. Secondly, she has had problems with irregular menstrual cycles and infertility. Her problems have been going on for quite a long time.

The Connection Between Antibiotics and Chronic Fungal Disease

Here is a brief explanation. When antibiotics are given, bacteria are killed. This includes good bacteria as well as bad bacteria. This causes an imbalance in your internal environment, your gastrointestinal tract, your sinuses, etc. Fungus that is already present will take advantage of the void left by the departing bacteria and grow to fill the vacancy. This is what we mean when we talk about fungal overgrowth. More fungi means more mycotoxins.

Fungi Produce Chemicals Called Mycotoxins

("myco"- fungus, "toxin"- poison). A fungal species can produce several mycotoxins and/or the same mycotoxin as another species. It is through these mycotoxins that fungi manipulate their environment to ensure a food source and their own survival. Some of these mycotoxins you may have heard of before: aflatoxin, ochratoxin, cyclosporin A and penicillin. That is right, penicillin is a mycotoxin. If you remember, Jennifer did state that she had received multiple courses of antibiotics when she was younger.

How Chronic Fungal Disease and Hypothyroidism Are Related

In my clinical practice, I have not seen a patient with chronic fungal disease that did not have some degree of decreased thyroid metabolism. Why does this occur? Here is what I have come to believe.

Your body works because all of its parts work together. If the lungs fail, oxygen does not get delivered, and energy in the form of ATP does not get made. If no ATP is made, the heart will stop beating. Certainly we can all agree that different parts of the body are dependent upon proper functioning of all of the systems of the body. The thyroid, adrenal glands, ovaries, testes, and immune system also share interdependence upon one another. When one of the members of this "endocrine-immune" group is over-worked or stressed, the other members are forced pick up the slack, so to speak.

Here is an example: When someone has a chronic fungal infection, it is almost always present in the gastrointestinal tract (dysbiosis). Dysbiosis allows proteins, viruses, bacteria and fungi to get into the tissues of the body, which would not ordinarily occur. Your immune system reacts to these foreign invaders by setting up an immune response (inflammation). As time goes on, the immune system becomes stressed from the chronic foreign invasion. Stress causes your thyroid metabolism to slow down and your adrenal glands to increase the production of cortisol. Increased cortisol production causes the release or production of inflammatory chemicals (cytokines) into the blood stream. This in turn causes more inflammation. Inflammation is the root of most all-chronic medical problems. You can probably see where I am going with this. The chronic fungal infection has to be stopped in order to break the cycle of inflammation.

Hypothyroidism is a recognized cause of infertility. The problem is getting traditional medical doctors to stop relying on laboratory work to diagnose hypothyroidism and start using their own clinical judgment. If it walks like a duck and talks like a duck, it probably is a duck.

Recommendations

Here are the recommendations that I made to Jennifer. I recommended that she begin on a daily natural anti-fungal such as olive leaf extract or grapefruit seed extract. I also recommended taking a daily probiotic to help restore her intestinal flora. Diet is essential to any successful treatment of chronic medical issues. I recommended an anti-fungal diet such as the Kaufmann Diet. I also started Jennifer on a prescription thyroid replacement hormone and recommended a regimen of vitamins and supplements.

Follow-up Visit

Jennifer presented to the clinic for a follow-up visit after four months. She states that her energy level has improved. She and her husband had just returned from white-water rafting and biking in Colorado. Jennifer strained her forearm paddling the river. She has also lost 23 pounds. Her husband came with her this visit. Seeing how much better his wife is doing has convinced him that he would like to start on the anti-fungal program as well.

Jennifer did not come into the office to be treated for chronic fungal disease. She came into the office because she felt bad and after many years, realized that traditional medicine was not helping her.

The best thing you can do for yourself is to be an active participant in optimizing your health. By far, the least expensive and most effective thing you can do is to change your diet. The Kaufmann Diet is the best place to start.

Blessings from Texas ,
Lynn Jennings, MD

What Can I Do If I Have Autoimmune Disease?

At the end of this book you will find the Kaufmann Lifestyle and the Kaufmann Diet in total. But, I want to give you some specific foods to avoid, specific foods you can eat and supplements you can take right now. Some of these things are becoming more common on the shelves of regular grocery stores. Others are best found at health food stores.

No matter what your health condition is, one principle to remember is that your gut has good fungus in it already, and it always will. We are not trying to eliminate it entirely. The objective is to keep from adding bad bacteria and fungi into the gut. When you eat the things you should avoid, you may be adding to these bad organisms into the gut, disrupting the balance between fungus and good bacteria that your body must maintain in order to stay healthy. In other words, while it is absolutely the best thing for maintaining balance to stay on the strictest form of this diet, it is highly challenging in our culture. There are so many SAD (acronym for the Standard American Diet) foods that contain the things you need to avoid.

In addition to the Kaufmann Diet, talk to your doctor about taking safe and inexpensive anti-fungal and probiotic supplements regularly. It is a more mechanical way of restoring and maintaining balance. Both together might really be what are needed.

Foods to Avoid

Immediately remove sugar, peanuts, corn, potatoes, most grains, mushrooms, pistachios, coffee and any foods containing them from your diet. For many of you, it may feel like I just took away all your birthday presents. These are your very favorite foods, I know! I am not a mind reader. Eating a lot of these SAD foods is why you are sick in the first place! If you are very sick, you need a radical change, which means you need to eliminate all of these things now. If not, you can work on them one or two at a time, starting with sugar and peanuts or corn. It will be a challenge. These foods are in over half of the things we eat. Some of us eat almost nothing but these foods. Say it with me this time: *This is why I am sick*!

Foods to Eat

The best meats to eat include grass-fed beef, buffalo, or lamb, wild-caught fish, and free-range, flaxseed-fed chicken. All of these meats are high in Omega-3 fatty acids. Eggs are also a great source of protein.

Nuts (not peanuts or pistachio nuts), green apples, berries, grapefruit and vegetables are generally safe as long as you remember that corn is not a vegetable—it is a grain. Fruits have sugars in them and can carry mold, so stick to those mentioned above with that caution in mind.

Supplements

Olive leaf extract is very good at eliminating fungus and mycotoxins. Curcumin is the best part of turmeric and is also a powerful anti-fungal.

Oregano oil is another powerful anti-fungal. When you start killing fungus in your body, it has a die-off reaction that feels like the flu. This, too, shall pass. Do not forget quality probiotics to restore balance in the gut.

CHAPTER 5

I Don't Have a Fungal Problem! I Am Suffering with Depression!

Depression as a chronic condition is a constant, heavy burden. It is a problem affecting every aspect of the lives of those who suffer from it. When depression strikes, hopelessness barely begins to describe your experience. The feelings of emptiness, anxiety and desolation do not cease with time but persist regardless of circumstances. You don't want to get out of bed in the morning, yet you do not want to go to bed at night. Moving through the day is like trying to run through water with weights around your ankles. Motivation is much like knowing the sun is there during a daytime thunderstorm, but it is invisible to you and you alone!

Depression affects not just you but those who surround you, and that only makes it worse for you. When you cannot function at all, you feel you are letting them down. Your coworkers, your husband or significant other, your children, your friends and anyone who remotely counts on you is going to have to get by until you recover, and you hate that.

If those people around you have never gone through depression themselves, it is especially difficult. You know they mean well when they say crazy things like, "Cheer up, buttercup," or try to relate by telling you how sad they were when their hamster died. You want to have patience for them, but you also want to thump their foreheads.

You know you ought to seek professional help, but you don't feel like you require a meeting with someone who treats crazy people. You are not crazy! You have two friends who suffer like you do; they have seen doctor after doctor and are now on handfuls of antidepressant medications and neither is improving.

Still, you understand that seeking medical advice can sometimes be lifesaving. Psychologists and psychiatrists see many patients who are not crazy but could benefit greatly from their help. The problem is, you are able to engage in life, and you worry about the drugs that will be prescribed to you. I do not blame you one bit. It is fair to tell a doctor that you feel that you may require his counsel, but not his prescribed drugs. Is that even an option? Do psychiatrists even counsel patients without handing them drug after drug?

What Is Depression?

Depression is almost like a mythical beast that is some weird combination of animals. There are obvious psychological and emotional components to depression, but it is also recognized as a medical problem with clinically observable symptoms. People who suffer with depression are often afflicted with unceasing feelings of despair, anxiety and hopelessness. These can be accompanied by feelings of restlessness or irritability. People with serious depression often have trouble sleeping at all or sleeping too much. Many lose interest in activities they once found pleasurable, such as work, hobbies or even time with good friends. Many experience fatigue, difficulty concentrating and problems with making decisions. Some people may lose their appetite, while others may overeat. In extreme cases, thoughts of suicide may occur. These symptoms can persist for weeks, months and even years on end without relief.

There are different varieties of diagnosable depression:

- Major Depression (clinical depression) is characterized by severe symptoms of depression.

- Persistent Depressive Disorder is characterized by a depressed mood that lasts for more than two years. Symptoms may become more intense or less pronounced during that time, but symptoms must last for two years to be considered persistent.

- Psychotic Depression is characterized by depression in addition to psychotic episodes, such as hallucinations, delusions, etc.

- Postpartum Depression affects mothers in whom classic signs of depression appear after childbirth. Sometimes it is immediately after and sometimes it begins several weeks or months after.

- Seasonal Affective Disorder is a type of depression brought on by lack of sunlight during the winter months.
- Bipolar Disorder is less common than other forms of depression. Sufferers oscillate between manic highs and depressive lows.

Why Are We so Depressed?

Each year in the United States, 6.7% of adults experience major depressive disorders. This represents over 16 million people with debilitating symptoms of depression. Once again, we see so many more women that men afflicted with depression. Women are 70% more likely to experience depression than men, which is why it was so important to me to devote an entire chapter to it.

The obvious question that comes to mind is, why are women so depressed? To answer that question, your doctor will likely try to assess your risk factors. Risk factors for depression, we are told, can be genetics, history of mental illness, traumatic or stressful events in your life and certain personality traits such as being self-critical, pessimistic and having low self-esteem. These seem to make sense, but are they enough to cause major depressive disorders?

We do know that depression is a disorder of the brain, and therefore, brain chemistry plays a role in the development of depression. MRI scans on depressed patients reveal physical differences in the brain when compared to the scans of those who are not depressed. [1] Hormones, too, can play a role. It is thought that changes in the way neurotransmitters function can play a role in mood and thus be a cause of depression. [2] This is a promising bit of information, but the most obvious follow-up question is, *what can cause altered brain chemistry and simultaneously disrupt your hormones?* Of course, the cause of those changes, you have been told, is currently unknown. "We just don't know," is a too-familiar theme in this book. Some of the most vexing and debilitating diseases, disorders and conditions entail or even focus on changes that current medical science simply cannot explain.

While many factors and causes may be implicated when it comes to depression, what your doctor will likely tell you is that we ultimately do not know what causes clinical forms of depression.

Treatment for Depression

Like most other illnesses, while the cause of depression remains unclear, there are many ways to treat the symptoms of depression. If you are diagnosed with clinical depression, there are two primary steps your doctor may take following the diagnosis.

Psychotherapy is a prevalent treatment for depression. Psychotherapy involves talking sessions with a mental health professional like a counselor, therapist, psychologist or psychiatrist. Psychotherapy can be very beneficial for people dealing with depression. Talking through the issues you are struggling with becomes an outlet for releasing the emotions of depression while giving you a method for coping with those emotions while going forward.

At the same time, many physicians will likely prescribe some form of antidepressant medication. These types of medications include selective serotonin reuptake inhibitors (SSRIs), serotonin-norepinephrine reuptake inhibitors (SNRIs), norepinephrine-dopamine reuptake inhibitors (NDRIs) and others.

You do not have to know what reuptake means. What you need to know is that all of these drugs serve one purpose: To restore the chemical balance in your brain...for 6 hours at a time and only if you continue taking medication. Often, antidepressant medications are prescribed in tandem with one another to find the right combination to combat symptoms of depression, but sometimes there are too many factors in play to get it right. You know the story: One pill is good, but three are better.

Furthermore, while these types of medications may aid in the abatement of symptoms of depression, they are not without side effects. These drugs are psychoactive, which means they do not just interact with your brain chemically; they interact with your brain's thought processes. Because of this, antidepressants are required by law to come with a black box warning, the strongest warning a prescription can come with. Many of these medicines increase the risk of suicidal thoughts and death.

You have probably heard the disclaimers on TV ads. It is enough to make you wonder why you would ever take such a medication. Yet, drug company advertisements are working well, and they are marketed widely. In fact, most people are familiar with the brand names of these types of medications, because advertisements for them litter the ad space provided by television shows, online markets, radio and print.

The saddest part of taking antidepressant medications for depression is their link to—you guessed it—depression and worse. So antidepressants can cause depression, just like one best-selling bone strengthening drugs can cause brittle bones. That, itself, is depressing!

Why Do Selective Serotonin Reuptake Inhibitors (SSRIs) Work?

As it turns out, no one quite knows how SSRIs actually work. This alone should frighten us. Based on its name, SSRIs work by stopping (inhibiting) the brain chemical serotonin from going up. That sounds simple enough. So is depression linked to low levels of serotonin? No, it is not, but they do work for some people. As is often the case with chemical medications, they tend to work, but our brightest and best tend not to know why. So we don't know why you have depression, but let's try a drug that might help, even though we don't know *why* it might help! Science at its best!

Let me offer this hypothesis on why SSRIs work in as few words as possible: They kill fungi that make poisons that are neurotoxic to our brain cells. In 2001, one of the most important research papers on an unknown property of SSRIs was published in the prestigious *Journal of Antimicrobial Chemotherapy.* [3] (Antimicrobial chemotherapy means chemicals that kills germs.) The doctors leading the research placed 4 different fungi into test tubes, then added the SSRI medications Zoloft, Prozac, Paxil, Celexa and Reboxetine to the tubes. The positive control was a known anti-fungal pharmaceutical drug used for killing toenail fungus called Sporanox.

These test tube studies clearly demonstrated anti-fungal affects of SSRIs. All 5 SSRI antidepressant drugs had fungicidal activity toward all species of fungus. This is important, because anti-fungal properties are twofold; they either stop fungus from metastasizing (fungistatin activity), or kill it completely (fungicidal activity). Even when the drug Sporanox could not kill one strain of fungus, each of the 5 SSRI antidepressants did! Zoloft and Prozac were the strongest fungus killers. In their discussion, these doctors stated that their discovery provided a rationale for the local treatment of fungal infections with formulas containing SSRIs. I do not, however, recommend you ever take these fungus-killing, antidepressant drugs to kill fungus. There are much safer ways to kill fungus than with antidepressant drugs. But it is fascinating to note, however, that the billion-dollar antidepressant drug industry might be so successful because their best selling wares kill fungus, and fungus can cause depression!

Following this breakthrough understanding of quite possibly why these antidepressants work, I can find absolutely no further studies to confirm this work. Selling pills is big business. Knowing why they work, on the other hand, is apparently not so important to anyone but you and me. Of course, this is terrible for those who suffer from depression and cannot figure out why, yet this one old research paper may help so many of you.

Now let us explore other links that may empower you to look at fungi and their poisonous mycotoxins as a possible cause of your depression.

Treating Depression: Big Business

Direct to consumer (DTC) marketing of pharmaceutical medicines is only legal in two developed countries, of which the United States is one. It is a practice that has developed into a multibillion-dollar industry. [4] Telling lay people to ask their doctor about potentially dangerous drugs that are only available with a doctor's prescription is a dubiously ethical practice that is only made possible by the mountain of cash pharmaceutical companies spend on ads.

In 2005, pharmaceutical companies spent $122 million on DTC advertising of antidepressant drugs. Their efforts were largely rewarded; it was estimated that over 27 million people in the U.S. were on anti-depressants in that same year, up from around 13 million five years prior. [5] As of 2013, it was estimated that 1 out of every 10 Americans was on anti-depressants—over 30 million people! [6] In 2011, sales of antidepressant drugs totaled over $11 billion. [7]

This amount of money tied up in the treatment of this medical condition is astounding. It is even more astounding that antidepressants can (and often do) cause depression or medical conditions that I deem are even worse than depression. In 2011, a *Psychology Today* blog finally gave a name to antidepressant-caused depression. It is called *Tardive Dysphoria*. [8] In the blog, they asked if antidepressants worsened the long-term course of depression. The very thought that antidepressants might be pro-depressants is staggering, but indeed for many people, they may be.

Despite the fact that all of these treatments may aid in the mitigation and masking of symptoms, even if they do work for some people, none of them work to address the root cause of clinical depression in the first place. In hopes of helping so many of you, let me set the stage for a tiny germ that I believe is intimately involved in altering brain chemistry and may exist at the very root of your depression.

In chapter two, you learned that many antibiotics are fungal mycotoxins. I believe that these poisons are fully capable of causing many health problems, not the least of which is depression. But how does a brain-toxic fungal poison get into your body in the first place? A past executive director of the Harvard Health newsletter wrote a headline in 2013 reading, *Infection, autoimmune disease linked to depression*. In this study that reviewed 92,000 people with mood disorders (depression), 22,320 had been treated for a serious infection before coming down with the mood disorder. [9]

Think about that for a moment. How would your doctor treat a serious infection? With an antibiotic, right? So, is the bacterium that caused the serious infection somehow to blame for the depression? Most likely not, although that is the direction that researchers will probably take. Rather, the more likely explanation (since antibiotics are mycotoxins and mycotoxins are fungal poisons) is that the antibiotics used to treat the infection are responsible for causing depression. Antibiotics are neurotoxic. Since they are linked with the most common forms of human cancer and a variety of other maladies, why could they not cause depression?

So, tell me, have you taken many rounds of antibiotics and now find yourself depressed?

Can Fungi Affect Mood?

As we have seen (and will continue to see in every chapter of this book), when a group of symptoms is declared to have an unknown origin, it is imperative to at least consider fungi and/or mycotoxins as an underlying cause. Currently, doctors don't do that, even though they are now being asked to by medical authorities. Fungi are everywhere and they do parasitize we humans. These facts make it a prime suspect, an assertion which is only made stronger by two facts. First, some mycotoxins, like penicillin, are neurotoxic. Second, our doctors study very little about the ability of fungal organisms and their poisons to affect human health. We have a significant problem in America that is very likely flying under the radar.

Clinical depression is a case in point. What we have is a set of symptoms that is prevalent in a population, whose symptoms are physical changes in the brain, but our brightest and best simply can not pinpoint the direct cause. Could it possibly be that a poorly understood fungal germ is responsible for those detectable changes in brain chemistry? Or could exposure to a neurotoxic fungal poison—via air, diet or medicine—be responsible for causing changes in the brain that lead to depression? You bet they could!

As examples, know that studies done on animals prove that fungal mycotoxins cause depression. In 2004, *The Journal of Veterinary*

Internal Medicine discovered that when a *Fusarium* mold mycotoxin called fumonisin was injected into healthy horses, it caused numerous symptoms including depression. [10] A few years later, in 2009, another prestigious journal, *Toxicon*, explored the same issue; could fungal mycotoxins induce or cause depression? This time, a known cancer-causing fungal mycotoxin (aflatoxin) was injected into study rats. (*It is of interest here to note that aflatoxin is widely used in research science to cause cancer in lab animals so that scientists can study cancer therapies or other medications*). To teach you just how potent and dangerous some of these fungal mycotoxins are, Toxicon researchers discovered that aflatoxin caused these rats to decrease feed intake and lose weight (a striking similarity to bulimia), get diarrhea and become depressed. [11]

Think about these two studies alone. As you have learned in previous chapters, our corn supply can expose us to both fumonisin and aflatoxin mycotoxins. We are eating small amounts of these mycotoxins if we are eating foods like cereals, breads, corn, peanuts, soy and other foods common in many people's diets. Are some of us more vulnerable to becoming depressed by that exposure? Or, consider the study subjects used. Scientists may scoff at studies that use animals and question how this carries over to humans. Ironically, their own peers do not use frogs or snakes or birds in these studies. They use mammals, because these are human-like. Horses, rats and we humans are all classified as mammals; each has a spine, grows hair and females breastfeed their young.

Yet, I find it so hard to believe that no (or very few, if they exist) psychiatrist or psychologist would understand that poisonous mold byproducts have been published in the scientific literature as causative agents of depression! They may not know it, but now you do. Think about your past exposure to mold and mycotoxins, be it in a moldy home or antibiotics in your past or perhaps a past problem with alcohol (itself the mycotoxin created by brewer's yeast). Each of these expose you to mycotoxins, and as you have just learned, mycotoxins can cause depression. This research is not unique when it comes to brain fungus.

Fungi and the Brain

The first question we should ask ourselves as we consider fungi a possible cause in depression and other brain symptoms might be this: Is it possible for fungi to gain access to the brain?

In *Principles and Practices of Clinical Mycology*, Dr. JR. Graybill describes fungal brain abscesses and fungal meningitis, a fungal infection of the area surrounding the brain. The different fungi that can gain access to this area of the brain include species of *Candida* (such as *Candida albicans*), *Cryptococcus neoformans*, *Coccidioides immitis*, *Histoplasma capsulatum*, *Blastomyces dermatitidis*, *Parracoccidioides brasiliensis*, species of *Aspergillus*, and species of *Zygomycetes*. [12]

You do not have to learn all those names. I include them to point out that the answer is not a tentative *yes*; rather, it is a resounding *YES*. While these sorts of infections are currently considered rare, they illustrate an important point; fungi can and do gain access to the brain.

But how? Dr. Graybill states, "Infection… occurs by direct contact… by inhalation… (or by) hematogenous (blood-borne) dissemination." This is what we talked about earlier in the book, that fungi can get in through breaks in the skin or inhalation, and now we learn that it can spread through the bloodstream. In fact, in a later chapter, fellow contributor C.C. Kibbler goes on to describe fungi being carried throughout the body via the blood stream. So, it is known that these fungi can disseminate via the blood stream, making their way to the brain.

With this in mind, is it possible that yeasts and fungi, once in the blood stream, can make their way to the brain, causing symptoms including those of depression? Is it possible that the vaginal yeast infection you experienced after rounds of antibiotics somehow disseminated throughout the body, finding its way to the brain? While many physicians may find this idea outlandish, looking at other ways fungi and their poisons affect the brain may shed more light on the subject.

Mycotoxins and the Brain

It has long been known and well-documented that fungal byproducts can have profound effects on the brain. Some studies have shown the effects of mycotoxins can mimic the effects of depression, which are found frequently in people exposed to water-damaged and mold-contaminated buildings. [13] This alone should be evidence enough to implicate fungus and mycotoxins in all cases of depression—a condition that our doctors will tell us has an unknown origin.

However, there are other well-known instances of mycotoxins influencing brain health. One of the most prominent cases, historically, of mycotoxins affecting human brain health is the case of the Salem Witch Trials. In this unfortunate event, girls were put to death under charge of witchcraft following a bout of hallucinations, spasms and other neurological symptoms. In that day, they did not know better than to blame supernatural evil. Today, it is generally assumed the girls were under the influence of ergot-contaminated rye. Ergot is another name for the fungus *Claviceps purpurea*. It can contaminate many types of grain, but rye is particularly susceptible. Ergot contains chemical components known to cause confusion and hallucinations. In fact, it was from ergot that the powerful, mind-altering drug LSD was first produced. Like many mycotoxins, ergot alkaloids can still contaminate our grain supply today.

There is actually a more commonly known mycotoxin that can have a very pronounced effect on mood. Many people use alcohol on a daily basis without knowing what they are consuming is actually a fungal byproduct. As previously mentioned, alcohol is the mycotoxin produced by brewer's yeast and is known to play a role in depression, both as a cause and as a means of self-medication for people who are depressed. When viewed through the lens of fungal influence on health, it should surprise no one that abuse of alcohol—a fungal toxin—can play a profound role in depression and mental health problems.

While these examples are well understood cases of mycotoxins playing a role in brain health—even causing what appears to be depression itself—the chances of your doctor implicating mycotoxins for your depression are low.

Do you recall the list in chapter two where I identified how toxic mycotoxins were to various parts of the body like the liver, kidneys and skin? One point was that mycotoxins were neurotoxic. This means that they are capable of damaging our nerve cells. Rarely would a doctor consider depression as a chronic mycotoxin poisoning, but that is the case with alcoholism, and it may be the case when you are exposed to other mycotoxins as well.

The mold *Penicillium* can grow in homes, and though its mycotoxin has saved many lives, penicillin has been known to be neurotoxic since 1945 and therefore fully capable of causing depression. At the right dose and with the proper delivery system, it was found to cause grand mal seizures and spasms and in some cases hallucinations in all age groups. Another commonly used antibiotic, amoxicillin, can also be neurotoxic. According to the 2011 *Physician's Desk Reference*, the side effects of amoxicillin may include agitation, anxiety, changes in behavior, confusion, convulsions, dizziness, hyperactivity and insomnia. So, the antibiotic you placed your child on is published as causing hyperactivity. Stop for just a moment and think about that! Doctor, why is my child hyperactive?

Think Back on Your Life

If you are suffering from depression, think about when your depression began. You might recall becoming seriously depressed after you were on several rounds of antibiotics or after living in a moldy home. Now, you have learned that fungi can infect nearly every tissue in the body via your blood stream, including the brain. Blood stream fungal infections are called systemic mycoses and—as you have now studied—may be the cause of your depression.

Fungi and mycotoxins are parasites that influence the behavior of their hosts. Their primary goal is to stay alive, and they do this by manipulating the host's chemistry to keep themselves well-fed. Many people who might perhaps be struggling with a fungal infection would likely crave the sort of foods necessary to keep those fungi alive. These are foods such as sugar, grain, corn, potatoes, starchy foods and alcohol. Without these foods, someone with a fungal infection likely feels crummy, almost flu-like. This represents such a small price to pay for starving these neurotoxic fungi.

Earlier in this chapter I italicized this sentence; *what can cause altered brain chemistry and simultaneously disrupt your hormones?*

We have discussed the ability of fungal mycotoxins to alter brain activity, but I want to just teach a little about these mycotoxins behaving in such a way as to disrupt your hormones. Our endocrine system includes hormone-producing organs within our bodies; pituitary, thyroid, parathyroid, adrenal, pancreas and the ovaries in females and testicles in males. The fungal mycotoxins known to disrupt these hormone producing glands are deoxynivalenol, or vomitoxin, T-2 Toxin and zearalenone. We are exposed to these through our food supply. One, zearalenone, is synthesized as a growth hormone and added to our beef and lamb supply. The FDA has shown that only trace amounts of the estrogen-mimicking product gets into us when eating, but I have to wonder how much of this product we are actually consuming. Because of scientific concern expressed by other countries (this hormone has been rejected for use as a growth promoter by The European Union), know that if you eat grass-fed and grass-finished beef, this hormone (also called Ralgro) likely is not in the meat. If you are concerned, always ask your meat provider to confirm that antibiotics and estrogen-mimicking hormones are not used in the meat he is selling you.

Now this is beginning to make more sense, right? You thought your pasta, bread or sugar cravings were not related to your depression. In many cases you must think again, but do not expect your doctor to understand this link unless he or she has studied this independently.

What Can I Do If I Am Dealing with Depression?

Since therapy is often effective for helping you cope with the thoughts that come when you are dealing with depression, seek a qualified counselor. If they recommend pharmaceuticals, ask if he or she will recommend a natural and safe treatment first like the one described in this book. These may or may not work to control your depression.

At the time of this writing, it is very unlikely that a mental health professional will consider the SAD (standard American diet) as a possible cause for your depression nor a change in diet as part of the solution. The Kaufmann Diet will definitely not hurt you, and it is possible that it could really help, as it tends to starve disease-causing fungi, so ask your mental health professional if you can try the Kaufmann Diet. If you alter your diet to match the Kaufmann Diet, there is a good chance you will make progress towards overcoming depression more quickly and more thoroughly. Even if it does not help your depression, it can help restore your gut microbial balance which can help with your overall health, and that alone may make you feel better.

Try the Kaufmann Diet for 30 days. Feeling less depressed? You have not cured your depression but you have finally figured out why you have suffered for so long. Without this knowledge, you would have likely spent the rest of your life battling and medicating.

Foods to Avoid
The Kaufmann Diet is explained in detail at the end of this book. Study it, try it and know that initially you may feel a bit worse as fungi tend to die-off and release toxins into your body as they starve.

Supplements to Try
Under no circumstances should you stop taking medications without your doctor's consent and assistance.

To minimize fungal activity, there are many safe supplements you can try. Again, since I do not know your medical history, please always check with your doctor before beginning an anti-fungal program. Three of my favorite supplements are Vitamin D3, curcumin and oregano oil. Taking a daily probiotic may help restore the balance in the intestines as you eliminate fungus.

St. John's Wort is a funny-named supplement that has been known to help some people with depression. Other supplements that have been studied for depression include 5-HTP, concentrated saffron, fish oil, rhodiola and SAM-e to name a few. Do not be intimidated by the names. They are all well-studied, considered safe and are readily available at your local health food store and online, but *PLEASE* work with your doctor to reduce the doses of your prescription medications as you begin to feel better. Do not try this on your own.

When it comes to depression, it is uncommon to find many doctors who will entertain the idea of using diet or natural supplements, so it may help if you work with a licensed/certified naturopath, herbalist, or other integrative specialist, and let them communicate with your doctor, so that he or she can decide if there are any interactions with medicines you may be taking.

This bears repeating: Under no circumstances should you stop any depression medicines you have been prescribed without your doctor's knowledge and assistance. Many of these medicines need to be tapered off slowly, if at all. Please do not mistake the suggestions in this book as medical advice. Work with your doctor and other licensed healthcare practitioners for diagnosing, prognosing, and prescribing medical treatments.

References:
(1) "Depression." *National Institute of Mental Health*, U.S. Department of Health and Human Services, www.nimh.nih.gov/health/topics/depression/index.shtml.
(2) "Depression (Major Depressive Disorder)." *Mayo Clinic*, Mayo Foundation for Medical Education and Research, 3 Feb. 2018, www.mayoclinic.org/diseases-conditions/depression/basics/treatment/con-20032977.
(3) Lass-Florl, C., et al. "Antifungal Properties of Selective Serotonin Reuptake Inhibitors against Aspergillus Species in Vitro." *Journal of Antimicrobial Chemotherapy*, vol. 48, no. 6, Jan. 2001, pp. 775–779., doi:10.1093/jac/48.6.775.
(4) "Direct-to-Consumer Advertising under Fire." *World Health Organization*, World Health Organization, 4 Mar. 2011, www.who.int/bulletin/volumes/87/8/09-040809/en/.
(5) "Antidepressant Use Nearly Doubles in U.S." *Consumer Reports*, www.consumerreports.org/cro/news/2009/08/antidepressant-use-nearly-doubles-in-u-s/index.htm.
(6) Rabin, Roni Caryn. "A Glut of Antidepressants." *The New York Times*, The New York Times, 12 Aug. 2013, well.blogs.nytimes.com/2013/08/12/a-glut-of-antidepressants/?_r=0.

(7) Dimond, Patricia Fitzpatrick. "Antidepressant Efficacy Called into Question." *GEN*, 1 Feb. 2010, www.genengnews.com/gen-articles/antidepressant-efficacy-called-into-question/3172/.

(8) Whitaker, Rob. "Now Antidepressant-Induced Chronic Depression Has a Name: Tardive Dysphoria." *Psychology Today*, Sussex Publishers, www.psychologytoday.com/us/blog/mad-in-america/201106/now-antidepressant-induced-chronic-depression-has-name-tardive-dysphoria.

(9) Skerrett, Patrick J. "Infection, Autoimmune Disease Linked to Depression." *Harvard Health Blog*, 17 June 2013, www.health.harvard.edu/blog/infection-autoimmune-disease-linked-to-depression-201306176397.

(10) Foreman, Jonathan H., et al. "Neurologic Abnormalities and Cerebrospinal Fluid Changes in Horses Administered Fumonisin B1 Intravenously." *Journal of Veterinary Internal Medicine*, vol. 18, no. 2, 2004, p. 223., doi:10.1892/0891-6640(2004)18<223:naacfc>2.0.co;2.

(11) Hussain, Salik, et al. "Toxico-Pathological Effects in Rats Induced by Concurrent Exposure to Aflatoxin and Cypermethrin." *Toxicon*, vol. 53, no. 1, 2009, pp. 33–41., doi:10.1016/j.toxicon.2008.10.008.

(12) Kibbler, C. C., et al. *Principles and Practice of Clinical Mycology*. Wiley, 2005.

(13) Campbell, Andrew W., et al. "Neural Autoantibodies and Neurophysiologic Abnormalities in Patients Exposed to Molds in Water-Damaged Buildings." *Archives of Environmental Health: An International Journal*, vol. 58, no. 8, 2003, pp. 464–474., doi:10.3200/aeoh.58.8.464-474.

CHAPTER 6

I Don't Have a Fungal Problem! I Have PMS, Endometriosis, or a Menstrual Disorder!

*We cannot erase time, but we can
take advantage of advances made over it.*

–D. Kaufmann

A few years ago, I recall seeing a book written by a woman that dealt with male prostate cancer. I recall thinking, "Why would I want to read a book about a male organ written by a woman?" Many of you might feel compelled to ask yourselves that exact question, especially as you read this specific chapter on female hormone and organ disorders, given that it is written by a male! Please don't disregard it, however, because I've learned tremendous lessons about female health problems from so many female patients and the doctors that referred them to me. The first few women I sat with decades ago told me that they were seeing me because they had sat with various doctors, including their own GYN doctors. They had all been told that prescription hormones were necessary to relieve their symptoms, and they simply did not want to take them. Somehow along the way, though, a physician referred them to me because I had helped their sister or one of their friends, hence their appointment with me. Maybe I can help you also, but how?

There is a theme you have probably already picked up in the book; I believe we must always "think fungus" for any medical condition that does not respond to traditional therapy. And so it was, while visiting a woman with sweat dripping off of the tip of her nose while talking to me, that I decided to stick with what had worked with many other medical problems that left so many people feeling helpless. I had a plan, and it might not work as well as it had on her friend, and it may not work for all cases of ___(fill in the blank)___, but what have we to lose by trying my plan? After all, it was safe while other plans were either unsafe or had failed.

Perhaps you are among the many women who go through a series of serious menstrual disorders only to have the whole rotation start over again. I have sat with so many women who mourn the loss of their reproductive system because medical science had no better answer for their endometriosis. Even worse are those who have come to accept that a hysterectomy is simply a normal part of life for a woman under 40. Although I do admit that sometimes these surgeries can fix your symptoms, unless the underlying cause has also been addressed and fixed, new symptoms will continue to plague you throughout your life. I believe that some female surgeries are often oversold as being normal procedures. But what are your options? I hope this chapter helps many of you, and *thank you for reading it*, knowing that it is a male who is busy typing away on the keyboard!

God put those organs in your body for a reason just like He placed our tonsils and appendix in their proper place for a reason. Antibiotics are sometimes necessary for infections in those tissues, but often they are surgically removed. When it comes to removing female organs, however, it is one thing for you to choose whether or when to start a family, and it is another thing to have that choice made for you! If you are one of those women and you have made peace with what you went through, I do not want to disturb that peace. I just want you to know that what you may learn in this chapter might have changed the course of action taken long ago. Science advances, and in doing so, we tend to shake our finger at it, but at the time you had the hysterectomy much of this information clearly was not known. *We cannot erase time, but we can take advantage of advances made over it.*

It is my job to give you information about these health problems that I have learned over the decades. Most likely you have not heard this information anywhere else. Armed with this information, you may be in a better position to make decisions that are best for you and your family. I give this same information to doctors at seminars, and the excitement begins for me when doctors learn new technologies to better help their patients. I have heard from several doctors recently that they have applied the information from my lectures on cancer to their patients' lives, and they are making a difference!

For those of you who have undergone a hysterectomy or similar procedure, this chapter may help you understand why you may have had so many health problems since. For those who are currently being told that a hysterectomy is your only choice, I am hoping this information opens your eyes to other possibilities that you and your doctor didn't know existed. If the information offers a safe and inexpensive approach that spares you both your uterus and your suffering, then I am thrilled!

Menstrual Disorders

Menstrual disorders encompass a variety of problems with a woman's menstrual cycle. If you have had them, you know the names. They include absence of menstruation (amenorrhea), painful cramps (dysmenorrhea), heavy bleeding (menorrhagia), infrequent menstruation (oligomenorrhea) and PMS (premenstrual syndrome). We will look at the related conditions together. We will also talk about the hormones that affect these conditions and endometriosis, a disorder that is affected by the menstrual cycle but goes beyond being merely a menstrual disorder. As you continue reading, I want you to know that your ovaries are an integral part of your endocrine (hormone-producing glands) system. Instead of including what a doctor does in defining the abnormality based on the excess or lack of blood, pain, or emotions associated with each disorder, let's try to understand the *cause of* each of these disorders.

Amenorrhea and Oligomenorrhea

Amenorrhea is clinically defined as going more than three months consecutively without menstruating or a failure to begin the menstrual cycle by the age of 15. Complications associated with amenorrhea include infertility and osteoporosis. Amenorrhea is typically caused by problems with the sexual organs and other glands that help regulate hormone function. Other causes include extremely low weight, eating disorders and excessive exercise. Some medicines can also cause amenorrhea.

Oligomenorrhea, or infrequent menstruation, is typically less of a concern. While it is an indication that something may be wrong in the body, there simply are not large numbers of women who are looking to fix this problem. Depending on what your doctor diagnoses as the underlying cause, contraceptive pills will likely be prescribed to help regulate your menstrual cycle.

Menorrhagia

Menorrhagia is excessive vaginal bleeding during menstruation. It is often accompanied by heavy cramping and sometimes symptoms of anemia such as shortness of breath and fatigue. There are a number of things that can cause menorrhagia including dysfunction in the ovaries, uterine fibroids or polyps or pregnancy complications. Certain medicines and intrauterine devices (IUDs) are also known to cause menorrhagia.

Other medical conditions or bleeding disorders may affect, cause or exacerbate menorrhagia as well. The medical community says that one of most common causes of menorrhagia is hormonal imbalance, and I believe that this assessment is absolutely correct. The complications caused by menorrhagia are anemia and severe, painful cramps (dysmenorrhea). To treat menorrhagia, doctors often prescribe contraceptives or other types of hormonal therapy along with iron supplements. What might cause hormonal imbalances?

Premenstrual Syndrome and Dysmenorrhea

PMS helps explain why one of the doctors' patients I was seeing became upset with me for starting our meeting on time! Seriously! Never had she had this happen in a medical setting, and she let me know in no uncertain terms that she will run late for her future visits. Interestingly as the nutritional approach began to work on her, she not only apologized for lashing out at me, but she began to come in on time! I didn't fully understand her anger at first, but I fully understand it now that I realized what was wrong with her.

Many women experience some symptoms of premenstrual syndrome (PMS) during certain parts of their monthly cycle, generally the days leading up to menstruation and during the following first few days. PMS encompasses a variety of emotional and physical symptoms. Emotional symptoms include appetite changes, anxiety, crying, depression, irritability, anger and the inability to concentrate. Physical symptoms include fatigue, headaches, fluid retention, bloating, joint and muscle pain, breast tenderness, acne, constipation and diarrhea.

For some women, the problems they experience due to PMS can be extreme and debilitating to the point that they interfere with their lives. Extreme symptoms of PMS are known as premenstrual dysphoric disorder (PMDD), which is pretty much a fancy way of saying really, really bad PMS, although what it describes is anything but fancy.

Despite how common PMS is, most mainstream medical practitioners do not understand its exact cause. The prevailing theory is that hormonal changes as part of a woman's monthly cycle play a role in creating symptoms. Women with serotonin deficiencies and depression are thought to be more at risk for experiencing symptoms of PMS than other women. These conditions are known to have hormonal roots, which is what makes it likely that hormones play a role in PMS as well. In extreme cases of PMS or PMDD, a doctor may prescribe anti-depressants or hormonal contraceptives.

Hormones: A Brief Overview

A unifying factor across most of these menstrual disorders is that hormones are known to play a role, so let us make sure we know what we are talking about. When we hear the word, *hormone*, we are most likely to start pushing away memories of being a moody teenager and the bodily changes that took place at that time in our lives. Because of that context most people have generally heard of the sex hormones, testosterone and estrogen. These hormones give men and women their respective, defining physical traits.

There are, however, a lot more hormones that we make other than testosterone and estrogen. Endocrinologists are physicians who study the hormone-producing glands within a person's endocrine system. Hormones are the chemical messengers in the body, and they play a variety of vital roles in our biochemistry. Hormones facilitate processes such as growth and development, metabolism, sexual function, reproduction and mood. We know that the sex hormones are produced in the testes of men and ovaries of women. Other organs within the endocrine system produce all other hormones. These include the pineal gland, pituitary gland, thyroid, thymus, adrenals and pancreas.

The Logical Question About Hormones

If hormonal problems are among the most common causes of menstrual disorders, the logical question to follow is, what could cause an underlying hormonal problem? There are a number of answers to that question, but sadly the etiology, or origin, of many problems rarely gets addressed in a routine, 30-minute visit to your doctor's office. Being handed a birth control prescription or supplemental hormones is, unfortunately, as good as it gets in most doctors offices. Honestly though, in your doctor's defense, what we are about to discuss is remote to him, so blame his education and educators, but not him.

If you are one of the women who experience menstrual disorders and have been quickly prescribed birth control or other hormonal therapies, you may be relegated to a lifetime of filling prescriptions. If this is you, you might be looking for relief from the financial burden, annoyance and sometimes-debilitating side effects of these drugs, not to mention long-term hazards. Perhaps I can help you, but again, please never stop taking prescriptive drugs on you own. An honest conversation with the doctor who prescribed these medications for you and letting him know that you are seeking change is always in order. Speak openly and honestly with him.

Hormonal Problems and Fungi

Is there a connection between fungi, mycotoxins and hormonal function? While most of the mainstream medical community would likely never blame fungi or mycotoxins for hormonal problems, any experienced farmer will likely tell you otherwise.

Much research has gone into the effects of mycotoxins on farming and livestock. Yes, you read that right. We spend more time and money studying the effects of fungi and mycotoxins on farm animals than on people. Why? Obviously, the impact of fungal mycotoxins on humans has been grossly overlooked, since we now know these fungal poisons can cause serious human illnesses. Rather than ever implicating them, it seems that new diseases and new drugs to treat them are an ever-growing field of pharmacology. Sick cows and chickens suffering from fungal mycotoxin-caused hormonal aberrations have a huge negative economic impact on the farming community. It is estimated that in the United States alone, mycotoxins cost the farming industry between $500 million and $5 billion each year. Sick women, however, suffering from these same disorders, pay doctors and pharmacies billions of dollars annually hoping for answers to their misery. *A sick chicken is never told by a veterinarian to try birth control pills.*

What Do Farmers Do?

Recall at the beginning of this book I taught that certain types of fungi are known to infest cereal grains. Because of conditions like drought, flooding or conditions in storage silos and during transportation, certain grains become vulnerable to fungal infestation. Many of the fungi that infest cereal grains produce mycotoxins which subsequently contaminate whatever the fungi land on or are eaten by.

Corn and other grains are staples of livestock feedlots. When grains have these disease-causing fungi in them and are fed to livestock, the animals can develop a variety of health problems. Known health problems in animals associated with mycotoxin ingestion include damage to vital organs, such as the liver and kidneys, increased incidence of disease and immune dysfunction, decreased reproductive capacity, vomiting, bleeding and a number of other problems, *including hormonal imbalances.* If fungal impregnated foods fed to livestock can cause these problems, might the same be happening to women with hormonal imbalances?

I went over this with you in chapter two, but it bears repeating one more time, especially in this chapter. If you have any doubt that fungi can wreak havoc on your hormones or your health in general, you must understand the following: Fungal mycotoxins in any mammal's environment, including their food, air or medications (recall that antibiotics are mycotoxins), including we humans, are known to cause mutations to our DNA, known to cause tremors and seizures, known to cause cancer, known to cause defects in a developing embryo, are poisonous to nerves, DNA, kidneys, liver, blood stream, heart and blood vessels, lymphatic system, skin and suppress our immune system, including blood cells. How I wish doctors knew this important information. In a word, yes; fungal contaminated food can cause the PMS, endometriosis and/or menstrual disorders you are having.

I say the word *contaminated* carefully here, because you might be surprised to learn that a known estrogen-disrupting fungal mycotoxin has not only been contaminating our food supply for centuries, but it is also being added to it on a regular basis.

What Might Be Causing All of These Female Hormone Problems?

There is little doubt that your mothers had far fewer health problems that were linked to hormone disruption 50 years ago than you have today. Let's try to discover why women today are being diagnosed with so many hormone disturbances that their mothers didn't seem to have. In doing so, you may find a few simple remedies available to every woman that may be of tremendous value to your recovery.

First, hormones are absolutely essential! They are good guys, but in excess they can easily become bad guys. Too many hormones being produced is a bad thing. It is well known that disrupted hormones contribute to many heath problems like diabetes. But estrogen disrupters, those unbeknownst to you or perhaps your doctor(s) that are elevating your levels of estrogen without your permission, may be making you very sick. These affect both men and women. Men with excess estrogen might find themselves with enlarged breasts or suffering from erectile dysfunction, but that is another entire book! Increases in a woman's estrogen levels may predispose her to a host of health problems including ovarian cysts, uterine fibroids, uterine cancer, breast cancer, infertility and possibly many more health problems. Women today suffer tremendously from hormonal imbalances. If we know that these symptoms are caused by elevated estrogen levels, why have our brightest and best never figured out the cause of elevated estrogen? The simple answer is that we have trusted chemical companies, who are run by good and sincere people I believe, but rarely is there oversight or vetting when a potent new chemical is accepted for use in our food supply. When it comes to what is elevating estrogen levels, there is no shortage of hypotheses floating around today as to why, and all are good and valid ones. But you didn't buy this book to to re-read old stories. You wanted updated information about why you have suffered so much.

Might I suggest that one of the reasons all of these hormonal health problems exist today is because of the 4 ton pink elephant in the exam room? There are estrogens being added to your food supply today that were not added when your mother was your age.

Certain poisonous fungal byproducts called mycotoxins are known to disrupt our normal hormonal flows. These are called *endocrine disrupters*, but they are also known as estrogen mimickers, since by mimicking real estrogen these can increase estrogen in our bodies. There are many estrogen disrupters, but let's try to hone in on those that didn't affect our mothers. For example, your mothers had dental mercury fillings, parabens in their cosmetics and deodorants and even ate foods like corn, each a potential endocrine disrupter. Fusarium is a fungal species that makes a mycotoxin called zearalenone, which is a known estrogen disruptor. For centuries, corn (maize) has been naturally impregnated by estrogen-disrupting hormones like those mentioned above.

If you're over 50 years old, you know that your mothers didn't drink plastic bottled water. We do. There is a chemical in certain plastics called bisphenol-A, or BPA. According to recent studies, we are exposing ourselves to hormone disrupters when we drink water out of plastic bottles containing BPA. Time magazine stated that nearly all of us now have BPA in our bodies, because we are so commonly exposed to plastic. Might plastic water bottles be causing all of your hormone problems? It's worth considering!

Without avoiding foods that become contaminated with the estrogen-mimicking mycotoxin zearalenone, both we and our mothers have still long been exposed to it. Several decades ago, a man-made form of zearalenone was approved by the FDA to use as a growth enhancer in cattle feed lots across America. As a matter of fact, a great research paper published in 2000 stated that at that time there were five hormones (progesterone, testosterone, estradiol-17β, zeranol, and trenbolone acetate) approved for implants in cattle in the U.S.A. But, it stated that these implants have been officially prohibited in Europe since 1989. [1] Of course, the first three of those are regularly made by we humans, but we don't make zeranol or trenbolone acetate.

The synthetic form of zearalenone is called zeranol (Ralgro), and it was a stronger version of the mycotoxin itself. If you are finding yourselves suffering from what you and your doctor feel are symptoms or diseases linked to hormone disruption, especially estrogen disruption, I think you need to know this. Mind you, the FDA cleared Ralgro as being safe in our food supply, but if you are consuming a lot of meats, dairy products (in which traces of Ralgro may occur) and grains, it may benefit you to take a few months off of bottled water and all dairy and meat products.

In 2017, a British Medical Journal study found that many diseases including, but not limited to, kidney disease, diabetes and cancer were associated with eating both red meat (including beef, lamb and pork) and white meat (including poultry and fish). [2] As we continue to genetically modify our food supply and add various chemicals to it, such a study doesn't surprise me. For many years now, scientists have been linking beef with cancer. I have to wonder if beef from cattle raised on a private farm without exposing the cow to added antibiotics/or estrogenic hormones has the same deleterious effect on our health that the meat from cattle exposed to these drugs is purported to have. Time will certainly tell and in the interim, you can choose to avoid this exposure to drugs and hormones in favor of meat that does not expose you to these contaminants.

Could a hidden toxin in our food supply be the root cause of the hormonal problems that cause menstrual cycle problems? After putting all of the pieces of the puzzle together, rewind back to your last doctor's visit; was there any mention of diet, specifically the presence of grains, bottled water or meat and dairy products in your diet? Has your doctor ever mentioned the words *estrogenic mycotoxin*? Likely not, because doctors would typically never suspect anything in your diet—let alone a fungal poison—of being the cause of a hormonal malfunction.

The fact remains that these fungal byproducts are in our food supply and may posses the qualities necessary to disrupt hormonal function. Again, let me reiterate that our FDA states that the amounts of Ralgro in our meat supply is insufficient to cause health problems, and I respect that. But we don't eat one piece of meat or dairy product daily. From our morning yogurt, to the cream in our coffee, to the bottle of water after our work-out, we are being exposed to hormone disrupters like never before, and I'm concerned that in some cases it this may be responsible for making you ill.

The take-away to remember is this: Farmers have a vested financial interest in keeping fungi and mycotoxins out of their livestock. Still, many of them unknowingly feed contaminated grains to their livestock which means the meat can become contaminated with these fungal mycotoxins also. Whether you eat grains and corn directly or through the meat you eat, you are likely exposing your own system to the mycotoxins inherent in these foods. A good immune system makes all the difference!

Polycystic Ovarian Syndrome (PCOS)

Polycystic ovarian syndrome, or PCOS, is not merely a menstrual condition. It is a systemic problem, which means it affects several organ systems in your body at once. Doctors often identify it when looking for reasons for the other menstrual disorders we have mentioned above. As of now, PCOS is one of the most common endocrine disorders among women of reproduction age.

PCOS is characterized as a hormonal problem, and it is. All men produce a certain amount of female hormones, and all women produce a certain amount of male hormones. This is normal. However, women with PCOS produce too many male hormones (called androgens) and that, it is thought, causes problems throughout their bodies. But is it?

PCOS affects approximately 5-10% of all females, and it has been diagnosed at all ages ranging from young girls 8-9 years of age up through women of menopausal age. Some of the more common signs and symptoms of PCOS are:

- Menstrual irregularities, including decreased number of menstrual cycles, irregular menstrual cycles (oligomenorrhea), or no menstrual cycle (amenorrhea) at all. Some women also experience heavy bleeding.
- Pelvic pain
- Accumulation of cysts on the ovaries
- Irregular ovulation
- Acne
- Thinning hair
- Excess hair growth on the face or body (hirsutism)
- Weight gain—60% of women with PCOS have weight management issues.
- Peripheral insulin resistance
- Infertility

Like many other systemic diseases and syndromes, what is labeled as a cause for symptoms does not go far enough. PCOS is a great example of this. When doctors say that PCOS is caused by an excess of male hormone production, and that abnormality is the underlying cause of these menstrual disorders, they are on their way to being right. They just have not addressed what is causing the excess of male hormone production that is causing what they are seeing!

This is much like a botanist teaching that the cause of leaves are branches, the cause of branches is this massive tree trunk and then stopping there without discussing roots. Most of us learned in elementary school that the first thing that a seed does is send out roots. It is essential that the botanist address the initial process instead of making it appear as though the trunk, branches and leaves appeared out of nowhere.

Something starts the process of excessive testosterone in a female, and it is not PCOS. The same is true of all physical diseases. As we just learned in the section on hormones, farmers know that fungi and mycotoxins wreak havoc on the hormonal systems of animals. They know that fungi and mycotoxins are sometimes the root causes of the diseases and syndromes that their livestock develop. Scientists who study mycotoxins have proven that these same fungal mycotoxins also affect humans on a cellular level.

One of the inherent dangers in medicine is that doctors observe an effect and believe that it is the cause. This happens far too often. PCOS may be a hormonal aberration in which excess male hormones are present, but could I respectfully add that zearalenone may play an important role in this disease also? In July, 2018, a medical journal stated that zearalenone in rats "…intensely manipulated the plasma hormonal factors and the level of gene expressions related to the polycystic ovary in rats, thus increases the risk of its progression." [3] I know that rats are not humans, but studies like these lend valuable information to causes of human diseases. Until doctors know this, the best that most women can expect is to be examined, have their blood tested for hormones, be told that they have cysts on their ovaries because their mother did (heredity) and then be handed diuretics and other medications. The logical question about what caused these cysts was never addressed. Not because the doctor was obnoxious, rather because he/she simply does not know this information.

If I were a female with PCOS, I would find a nutritionally-oriented healthcare provider that I was comfortable with and inquire about safe anti-fungal supplements like borage oil and evening primrose oil. Also, I'd think of a diet specifically aimed at nutritionally satisfying me while simultaneously staving fungal parasites like those that make mycotoxins. Such a diet does exist; keep reading.

Endometriosis

Endometriosis is a painful disorder in which the tissue that normally lines the uterus (known as the endometrium, or endometrial tissue) grows outside the uterus. Your body was not designed for this to happen. If you have endometriosis, when you are menstruating, these tissues growing outside the uterus undergo the same changes as the tissues inside the uterus where they belong. Your body has a simple process for dealing with the tissues inside the uterus, but it has no such process for when these tissues produce waste outside the uterus, and it can mistake this for an invasion or infection.

Like PCOS, endometriosis is a systemic problem that involves the bowel, ovaries and tissue lining the pelvis. It is as if a cyst-filled sac network has engulfed these organs. It can cause pelvic pain, painful periods, pain during sexual intercourse, painful bowel movements, painful urination and heavy bleeding during your period or between periods. Endometriosis can also cause tissue scarring. Women with endometriosis typically have a harder time becoming pregnant.

While the exact cause of endometriosis remains unknown, there are some ideas about what may contribute to its development. It is thought that retrograde menstruation, which is menstrual blood containing endometrial cells flowing back through the fallopian tubes, can implant endometrial cells in the pelvic cavity. These cells attach, thicken and grow on a monthly cycle the way the endometrium does in the uterus. Other potential causes include immune system disorders, surgical procedures, and a back flow of endometrial cells into the lymphatic system.

Hormonal therapies may help relieve some of the symptoms of endometriosis, but the relief often stops upon discontinuing treatment. In the most extreme cases, total hysterectomy is recommended. This has likely happened to thousands of women who thank God that they are out of their pain after a complete hysterectomy. I fully understand that! With drugs and surgery so available and so heavily used, why should we research the cause? Because understanding what started a disease will help you to better understand how to stop a disease.

Is Endometriosis a Misunderstood Fungal Infection?

While shopping in a remote bookstore in Austin, TX one afternoon several years ago, I noticed that the owner had all of his books in a database. I inquired if he had any books on mycology, or the study of fungus. Indeed, he had one for $25. The book was dated 1932. I was thrilled, because generally these are the best books for finding hints about the causes of disease from a time when drugs weren't so accessible; these books were written long ago when doctors, in my humble opinion, had more interest in being scientists than in erasing symptoms 4-6 hours at a time with a prescriptive drug.

Fungous Diseases, by Dr. Harry Jacobson, MD, recalled the case of a young Mexican woman who presented in his office with lower abdominal pain. The pain began at age 15 shortly after she was married to a much older man in Los Angeles. While she admitted promiscuity, the young woman had never been treated for any sort of venereal disease. The pain progressed to the extent that she was operated on, during which time it was discovered that, "…there were extensive adhesions between the pelvic organs and loops of small intestines… Both (fallopian) tubes and the right ovary were destroyed by the inflammatory process and the broad ligaments were extensively infiltrated."

Post surgically, a fistula (an abnormal passageway) containing pus developed in the surgical wound. This wound was drained and cultured.

What was cultured from the wound became her diagnosis, because the word "endometriosis" had yet to be invented. On the petri dish grew *Coccidioides immitis*, a disease-causing fungus known to infect human beings. The young woman was treated with colloidal copper, a safe and natural anti-fungal agent. She went on to make a full recovery of her wound and her illness. Her presenting disease was reversed with a petri dish and anti-fungal treatment.

What Dr. Jacobson described above is eerily reminiscent of what is called endometriosis today, but that was not what the doctor diagnosed the young woman with. Instead, he discovered that she had a fungal infection. Different species of *Coccidioides* fungi are generally found in semi-arid regions around the world, including Mexico and California. As a side note, Eastern America has different fungal diseases called histoplasmosis and blastomycosis due to the different fungi that inhabit the soils in that area. *Coccidioides* fungi is also the known cause of the disease Valley Fever which is difficult to diagnose. Just so you know, *Coccidioides* lung fungal infections have also been misdiagnosed as lung cancer.

What do these things have to do with each other? Putting the pieces of the puzzle together, could it be that endometriosis is, in fact, a fungal condition? We know that fungal infections are difficult to diagnose and can often mimic other conditions. As is the case with many diseases, doctors may rush to diagnose a condition, hoping to help a patient as quickly as they can, but often that rush excludes ruling out fungus as the cause. Talk to your doctor about this. I have learned that all doctors took courses during medical school in microbiology. Unfortunately, bacteriology and virology took precedence of the study of fungus, called mycology. Help your doctor renew his interest in this field!

It isn't just these strange sounding diseases that play a likely role in endometriosis. A little knowledge of the physical appearance of the *Candida* yeast in our guts could help explain how the cells that grow into extra-uterine endometrial tissue get out of the uterus in the first place. If you were to look at the yeast in the gut of an infant, it looks non-threatening. Its shape is characterized by gentle curves, kind of like a camouflage pattern of clouds. When it begins to overgrow, however, it looks spiky and more threatening. *Candida* yeast, fully capable of causing illness, can penetrate tissues, allowing contained systems to lose containment. If it pierces the uterus, endometrial cells can escape. When they escape, they take up residence in parts of your body where they do not belong and you may end up diagnosed with endometriosis, the root of which may be caused by fungus.

Hormones Are so Often the Key

Menstrual disorders have increased simultaneously with the standard American diet which has earned the acronym SAD. Do we really expect to eat 6 month old preserved food in boxes and cans and enjoy great health? Why are our healers not teaching us that this is not nourishing?

We have demonstrated how mycotoxins and fungus affect hormone production in animals and in people, as well. The female reproductive system is the part of your body that is most obviously connected to your hormones. A healthy diet lends to healthy immune and hormone systems. Disruptions in hormone levels can cause many problems.

When hormones are out of balance, a number of things can go wrong with your reproductive system. Doctors often treat them in isolation until there is a reason to treat them together, and that reason usually comes after you have been suffering for a long time from multiple symptoms in multiple systems of your body. Since menstrual disorders may be troublesome signs of deeper problems that are eventually said to be caused by a syndrome like PCOS or an observable condition like endometriosis, it makes perfect sense to, at the very least, consider and rule out hormone disruptors like fungal mycotoxins as a possible cause. These hormone disruptors enjoy ease of entrance into our bodies via HVAC systems in our homes and in our food and medication supply, yet physicians remain largely unaware.

Therefore, you may wish to consider treatment options that include a change in diet and lifestyle. The Kaufmann Lifestyle and Kaufmann Diet, both itemized later in this book, are specifically formulated to help your body meet and overcome these challenges.

References:
(1) Briefings, Fri & Doyle, Ellin. (2018). Human Safety of Hormone Implants Used to Promote Growth in Cattle.
(2) Etemadi, Arash, et al. "Mortality from Different Causes Associated with Meat, Heme Iron, Nitrates, and Nitrites in the NIH-AARP Diet and Health Study: Population Based Cohort Study." *Bmj*, Sept. 2017, doi:10.1136/bmj.j1957.
(3) Abbasian, Nakisa, et al. "Molecular and Biochemical Evidence on the Role of Zearalenone in Rat Polycystic Ovary." *Toxicon*, vol. 154, 2018, pp. 7–14., doi:10.1016/j.toxicon.2018.07.022.

Polycystic Ovarian Syndrome (PCOS) Case Study and Solutions

This is an excellent example of how symptoms in unrelated systems can be traced back to fungi and mycotoxins as a root cause. As you read through this, see if you can identify where the problems Tina is experiencing began.

By Lynn Jennings, M.D.

For legal purposes I must always give this disclaimer: This case study is for educational purposes only. I am using it to show you how a typical patient presents and the things I consider when I make a diagnosis. The patient's name has been changed to protect her identity. I practice integrative/alternative medicine, and my recommendations for treatment are often considered outside traditional practice. It is not my intent to criticize or denounce traditional medicine. I am merely providing an alternative opinion. Most importantly, the information provided here should not be used as a substitute for an examination and treatment by a licensed health care provider.

Presenting illness:

Tina is a 17-year-old female who came to the clinic with her mother and younger sister for treatment of back and neck pain. She had been involved in a motor vehicle accident three weeks before her visit. Tina said that she does not have any recollection of the accident. At the time of the accident, Tina was taken to the emergency room for evaluation. In the emergency room, she underwent diagnostic imaging and was released.

Tina reports that she has constant, sharp aching in the muscles of her neck. She is also experiencing episodes of dizziness, which are unpredictable and not associated with any particular action or movement. She also reports a sharp, aching pain in the muscles of her lower back but no radiating pain or numbness in her legs or feet.

Past medical history:

Tina has exercise-induced asthma and a history of multiple allergies. Tina has been diagnosed with polycystic ovary syndrome (PCOS), the most common female endocrine disorder. Polycystic ovary syndrome gets its name from the multiple, fluid filled sacs/cysts that are often found on the ovaries of affected individuals. Although the cause is unknown, it is recognized that women with PCOS have a hormone imbalance. She has also been diagnosed with Acanthosis nigricans (AN), a skin condition characterized by dark, velvety skin in body folds and creases. It frequently affects the lateral and posterior neck, armpits, and groin, although it can also be seen in other areas of the body.

Medications and allergies:

Tina is on metformin and Loestrin for polycystic ovary syndrome (PCOS). Tina has an albuterol inhaler which she uses as a rescue inhaler. She takes Zyrtec daily and receives weekly injections for her allergies. Tina reports no known drug allergies. She states that she is allergic to grass, trees, weeds, cats, horses and pollen.

Social history:

Tina is a high school student. She lives at home with her parents. She does not smoke tobacco or drink alcohol. Tina does not exercise.

Review of symptoms:

Since her accident, she is having problems with headaches. Tina reports that she has problems with gastric acid reflux. She has been told that she is pre-diabetic.

When Tina was 2 years of age, she suffered from pneumonia which was treated with antibiotics.

Tina reports that when she was in junior high, after exercising she would experience dizziness and her skin would turn "bright red". She also reports that when she has been in the sun and then goes into a pool, she develops hives. The hives last for less than 30 minutes and are not associated with shortness of breath. Her doctors have labeled this problem urticaria.

Tina reports excessive hairiness, and she has been told that this is the result of increased production of male androgens. She also suffers from skin tags.

Tina says that she sleeps all the time and she also takes naps every day. Her mother reports that Tina does not snore.

Tina reports that her menstrual cycles are irregular. She states that she is taking the Loestrin to help regulate her menstrual cycles.

Tina suffers from pre-menstrual migraines.

Family history:
Tina's family history is significant for diabetes, migraines, hypertension and arthritis. There is no family history of polycystic ovary syndrome or acanthosis nigricans.

Physical exam:
Blood pressure:115/75 Pulse: 91 Weight 214 lbs. Height: 5'8"

Tina was noted to have scalloping of her tongue.

She was also noted to have hyper-pigmentation of her posterior and lateral neck with scattered skin tags.

Her elbows show very dark plaques that raise above the surface of her skin.

Tina was also noted to have tightness and spasm in the muscles of her back and neck.

The remainder of her physical examination was unremarkable.

Discussion:
Traditional medical treatment for PCOS includes using medications to regulate the menstrual cycle in the form of birth control pills and metformin. Metformin is a first line medication for Type 2 diabetes. Although it has several mechanisms of action, it is thought to lower

blood sugars by decreasing the production of sugar by the liver and reducing insulin resistance. Other treatments for PCOS include treatment for hirsutism with spironolactone or topical Vaniqa.

The most common causes of acanthosis nigricans are conditions in which there are increased insulin levels or insulin resistance, which leads to increased circulating insulin levels. The increased insulin levels stimulate the formation of skin plaques and skin tags.

The conditions most often associated with insulin resistance are Type 2 diabetes, obesity, and polycystic ovary syndrome. Certain medications may also be associated with increased circulating insulin levels, including oral contraceptives, steroids, and of course, insulin. Acanthosis nigricans may be inherited, although this is not the case for Tina.

There is no specific treatment for acanthosis nigricans, but treating the underlying causes of the increased insulin resistance may cause the skin discoloration to fade. Direct from the Mayo Clinic website, the first two recommendations are losing weight if you are overweight and making dietary changes, such as cutting back on your intake of sugar and starches. However, the website also suggests that medications such topical Retin-A and oral isotretinoin (Accutane) as well as dermabrasion and laser therapy may be helpful.

So why have I chosen Tina as a case study? She is a millennial. In spite of all of the advancements in medicine these children are unlikely to live as long as we do or even be as healthy as we are.

As a group, these children have been consuming processed foods, conventionally farmed foods (i.e., confined animal factory operations), and genetically modified foods for most of their lives. High fructose corn syrup, other corn products and peanuts are in most processed foods. Most have received or will receive the 49 vaccinations recommended by the CDC by the time they are 18 years of age. (If you do not include the human papilloma virus series, it would only be 46.) Many in this generation consider using a microwave oven as cooking. Does it surprise you that this generation of individuals would seem to be less healthy than their baby boomer grandparents?

I feel as though I should add a few words about their generation X parents. One of the things that generation X and the millennials share in common is that they have been the recipients of serial antibiotic use for otitis media, strep throat and acne, just to name a few.

One of the side effects of taking antibiotics is fungal overgrowth. When you are given an antibiotic, the idea is to kill the bad bacteria that are causing the infection. Unfortunately, antibiotics are non-specific; they will kill off good bacteria as well as bad bacteria. Fungi are opportunistic; when good bacteria are killed by antibiotics, this leaves a vacancy and no competition for space or food. Fungi that are present will grow to fill the vacancy left by the bacteria. In some cases, this will show up as a vaginal yeast infection or even thrush (candida of the mouth). However, most of the time we are not even aware that there is a problem. Chronic fungal overgrowth is more often insidious, and it can be present in every tissue in our body including our sinuses, lungs, prostate and gastrointestinal tract. Gastrointestinal fungal overgrowth is known by several names: leaky gut, dysbiosis or intestinal hyper-permeability.

Leaky gut is associated with several problems. When present, our gastrointestinal tract loses some of its ability to absorb nutrients properly from foods. This can lead to malnutrition as well as relative vitamin deficiencies. When dysbiosis is present, the normal barrier lining of the GI tract is disrupted at a microscopic level. The spaces between the cells lining the intestines get too large. This allows toxins, protein molecules, bacteria, and fungi (yeast) to enter into the body and bloodstream that ordinarily would not. When these protein molecules, bacteria and fungi enter the tissues surrounding the intestinal tract, the immune system recognizes these as foreign invaders and begins to attack. The immune response to the perceived foreign substances is essentially an inflammatory response (inflammation). Chronic fungal overgrowth is associated with chronic inflammation. Fungi manufacture chemicals which are called mycotoxins. Mycotoxins are chemicals that fungi use to manipulate their environment and assure a source of food in the form of sugar (glucose). What may be surprising to you is the fact that mycotoxins can be associated with most human health problems. The more fungi present, the more mycotoxins present.

With regards to diabetes and peripheral insulin resistance, the *Aspergillus* mold mycotoxin, aflatoxin B1, inhibits the breakdown of sugar and glycogen (stored form of sugar in the liver). When the ability to break down sugar is inhibited, the sugar remains in the bloodstream at elevated levels. Elevated blood sugars are associated with diabetes Types 1 and 2. Aflatoxin is commonly found as a contaminant of corn.

Streptozotocin, also a mycotoxin, can cause decreased insulin sensitivity (peripheral insulin resistance) which is found in diabetes Type 2. It can also damage the pancreas, where insulin is produced, leading to diabetes Type 1.

Ochratoxin, a mycotoxin commonly found on peanuts, corn, wheat and other grains, is associated with depletion of glutathione (GSH) stores in our body. Low glutathione levels are associated with insulin resistance. Diabetics typically test low for GSH.

As we see above, chronic fungal infection can be associated with diabetes Type 1 and Type 2. Could it also be associated with polycystic ovary syndrome (PCOS)?

PCOS is primarily characterized by excess production of male sex hormones (hyperandrogenism), insulin resistance and chronic menstrual irregularities. Increased insulin levels change female hormone metabolism towards androgen dominance, which means that testosterone becomes more dominant than estrogen. Excess androgens increase levels of free fatty acids that inhibit liver detoxification and inhibit skeletal muscles from using glucose. These metabolic pathways create a vicious cycle of elevated insulin that is fed by—and feeds—androgen formation. The increased insulin levels found in PCOS cause the ovaries to manufacture excessive amounts of testosterone.

Hirsutism is defined as the presence of excessive hair in androgen-dependent areas of a woman's body. Testosterone stimulates hair growth and increases hair size and pigmentation. This is a real problem for women with PCOS.

The good news is that a study in 1996 compared three of the most common treatment regimens for hirsutism in women with PCOS. Ketoconazole, an anti-fungal drug (as the "alternative" treatment), was compared with an oral contraceptive (birth control), Cyproterone (synthetic, anti-androgen hormone) and spironolactone (diuretic). Ketoconazole was the most effective in decreasing hirsutism and decreasing free testosterone levels.

What? A medication that kills fungus can help decrease hirsutism? Makes you think, doesn't it?

Conclusion and Treatment

Tina's case demonstrates the development of serious chronic medical disease in a very young person. With the diagnosis of PCOS, she is at increased risk of developing other serious medical problems such as high cholesterol and triglycerides, cardiovascular and heart disease, diabetes, sleep apnea and endometrial cancer. This is serious.

I believe that she has had chronic fungal overgrowth since a very early age, possibly dating back to her problems with pneumonia. Add to this your typical American diet with far too much sugar and highly refined carbohydrates. Add also no exercise or greatly reduced exercise. This is a recipe for disaster.

What would I recommend for Tina? First and foremost, I would recommend a changed diet! If anyone needed an anti-fungal diet, this young woman does. I recommend the Kaufmann Diet. I also recommended that she begin taking a natural anti-fungal, such as olive leaf extract or oil of oregano, and probiotics daily. As part of the treatment for her muscle spasm and pain, she will begin an exercise program designed to strengthen her core musculature. She needs to exercise, which will help reduce her insulin resistance.

At present, I would continue her metformin. This is one of the few medications for the treatment of diabetes that is not associated with weight gain and has been shown to be helpful in lowering blood glucose. Natural supplements that work similarly in the body include berberine, bitter melon and chromium picolinate. I would also recommend that once these other measures have been put into place, she should discontinue her birth control pills and let her natural hormone balance re-establish itself.

One of the concepts I would like for everyone, including health professionals, to understand is this: You need to look for the cause. Taking medications to treat a symptom of a disease does not ultimately resolve the underlying medical problem. In the words of a very astute physician, "You can not medicate your way out a disease you have behaved yourself into." Our children and grandchildren have received the best that modern medicine can provide. It is only with education about the benefits of diet and exercise that the promise of a healthy future will be theirs.

Thank you, Dr. Jennings!

What Can I Do If I Have These Conditions
Most importantly, find a doctor like Dr. Jennings, who has been exposed to the knowledge of how fungi and mycotoxins are the underlying cause for all these seemingly unrelated groups of symptoms across your body. Remember that diagnosis and treatment is best done by someone with complete training who will know how to consider your current medications. Do not stop taking medications you have been taking without talking to your doctor.

At the time of this writing, you might discover that finding a doctor who knows fungus and mycotoxins is a lot like finding a needle in a haystack when the haystack covers the entire US and there are only a handful of needles. That is okay. You can talk with your doctor now about starting on the Kaufmann Diet, which is specifically formulated to reduce your exposure to foods that are contaminated with fungi and mycotoxins, reduce your intake of sugar and other sweeteners that feed fungi and increase your intake of uncontaminated foods and foods that help eliminate fungi and mycotoxins that are already in your body.

Severe problems: If you have endometriosis or PCOS, and you are experiencing symptoms in other systems of your body, you need to make radical adjustments in your lifestyle and diet. Please immediately consider talking to your own doctor about declaring a sugar fast. If approved, make it a game with yourself to see how long you can go without sugar. You can build in a cheat day no more than once a week as long as you keep it to a bare minimum. Also eliminate mushrooms, corn, potatoes, peanuts and grains completely. That includes anything made from corn, peanuts or grains. Stop drinking coffee as well. If the diet has been approved, talk honestly with your doctor about adding some naturally anti-fungal and probiotic supplements to your daily routine. There is a list of these in the last chapter.

Tell yourself that your very life depends on how well you do these things, because it truly may. Keep a positive attitude, knowing full well that you may feel a bit worse initially, but within a short period of time, the old you might reappear! Where has this you been?

Moderate problems: If you have endometriosis or PCOS with no other systemic symptoms, or you have more than one of the menstrual disorders, you may not need to be so radical. It will not hurt you, so if you are inclined to make a radical change, after speaking with your own doctor, go for it. However, you can work towards it slowly.

The more you can stick to a few simple diet restrictions, the sooner you can expect results.

Minimal problems: If you have only one of the menstrual disorders and no other symptoms anywhere else in your body, you may be catching this early, and that is very good. Taking a radical approach may get you better faster. However, you might get back to health without having to be so drastic right now. Focus primarily on adding supplements. This may help neutralize any fungus that has accumulated in your body. Begin to eliminate the detrimental food items one at a time to build up to the point of eliminating or drastically reducing all of them. I do not know your health history, but your doctor does. Always get approval from him/her before you begin a new diet or exercise program.

CHAPTER 7

I Don't Have a Fungal Problem! I Just Have a Skin Problem!

I had been coming to Dallas from Los Angeles for over a year to assist Dr. David Weakley in his ever-expanding dermatology practice, and it was time for a permanent move. He loved what he was seeing in the patients he referred to me. So in 1987, we packed up our family and relocated to Dallas, Texas. His toughest patients, those who were resisting traditional approaches like ultraviolet boxes, tar shampoos and cortisone shots, became my clients. With his full permission, I would educate each of these patients on my fungal hypothesis. I will share the program that we implemented with you toward the end of this chapter.

As you may have guessed by now, I believed that fungus had much to do with their miserable skin conditions. I am not talking about obvious fungal skin conditions like ringworm and nail fungus. Armed with anti-fungal drugs, Dr. Weakley easily took care of those. I am talking about the people like you, who were suffering from strange skin problems, people that had been to several doctors trying to figure out what their problem was, to no avail. Regardless of how long they had been suffering from the condition or the severity of it, it seems like their condition never quite went away.

Skin problems are not only irritating; they can also be quite embarrassing. Most of the time, an unsightly rash accompanies the irritation. There is something about seeing a rash on someone that just screams to those around you, "Stay away!" When the rash is in an intimate area, it affects our partners as well.

At his dermatology practice in Dallas, after carefully explaining the program to each one of his patients and with his full permission and approval of each case, he and I would put them on a course of treatment and scheduled a follow-up visit 14 days later. I recall Dr. Weakley requesting a box of Kleenex in each exam room because of the many tears that flowed when many of his "cause-unknown" patients went their first week without traditional medications and without their skin flaring up.

So many of you reading this book are in the same boat that those patients were, because your dermatologist, urologist, internist, general practitioner, psychiatrist, orthopedist, gynecologist or neurologist does not understand fungal disorders and how very, very common they actually are. Who can blame them? Even today, medical education is void of mycology, or the study of fungus. In 2007, the respected American Academy of Microbiology stated, "Fungi are the cause of many outbreaks of disease, but are mostly ignored. Fungi can cause a number of life-threatening diseases…. Many people, scientists among them, are largely unaware." *Houston, we have a problem!*

As we enter this chapter, know that hundreds of Dr. Weakley's patients learned that their symptoms did not have an off/on switch, but they did have a "rheostat," or volume control, wherein they could adjust their symptoms up or down, depending upon their own lifestyle choices. It is my hope that you, too, find your own rheostat control somewhere within the pages of this book.

The Largest Organ

The skin is quite a remarkable part of the human anatomy. It is the largest organ in the body, encapsulating all the other systems that comprise your physical being. As such, it plays many important roles. It is our first line of defense against all environmental threats to the body; this makes the skin a critical part of the immune system. It provides protection from would-be microbial invaders, heat, cold, the sun's ultraviolet rays and water. It provides an environment where the biochemical processes that support life can take place. It provides the platform for our sense of touch. This makes the skin an important part of the way we orient ourselves in the world. All in all, the skin's role in life and health is as important as any other organ system in the body.

The skin has the added role of being an important part of one's appearance. Vibrant, healthy-looking skin is seen as a marker for youthfulness, health and vitality. Particularly for women, maintaining the youthful appearance of your skin is an important part of your self-image. Marketers and cosmetic manufacturers are not blind to this reality, and to that end, they spend many millions of dollars every year on marketing their wares to women, promising vibrant, clear skin. And their efforts are not going unrewarded. Huffington Post reported in 2013 that women spend upwards of $430 billion on beauty products each year. Imagine what the number is today!

The great irony is, while healthy skin is thought of as a sign of overall health and wellbeing, many of the products sold to us with the purpose of making our skin more lustrous are actually detrimental to your health. A large percentage of the skin products—many of which absorb through the skin and into the bloodstream—are loaded with toxic chemicals. Many are linked to serious health problems, including cancer. Products such as soaps and lotions often contain harsh foaming agents such as diethanolamine, triethanolamine and sodium lauryl sulfate; all of these chemicals have been implicated somehow in cancer. Other cosmetics contain methyl-, ethyl-, butyl- and propyl- parabens. All are used as preservatives and have been found in breast cancer tumors.

So while we are covering our skin in products with the goal of appearing healthier, it is likely we are not doing our health any favors in the long run. Many of these chemicals break down our skin tissues on a microscopic level over time. The more your skin breaks down, the more susceptible it is to a microbial invasion.

The intent of this chapter is not simply to berate the cosmetic industry or to point fingers. However, if skin health is so important that we seek to preserve it, we should ask ourselves the same question we should ask with anything pertaining to our health: What is the underlying cause of the problems we experience, in this case with our skin? Perhaps I can shed some light on the subject.

Fungus and the Skin

An irony with the skin is that its job is to protect us from disease-causing microbes, but it has no way to kill them. That is why I have mentioned again and again that fungi residing on our skin are one way that they get into our bodies. It is no secret that fungal infections of the skin are common. Many people have experienced fungal infections like ringworm, jock itch, athlete's foot or topical *Candida* yeast infections. Generally, these are assumed to be superficial infections, and while annoying and perhaps embarrassing, usually they are treated with over-the-counter anti-fungal medications or topical treatments, and/ or prescription anti-fungal drugs.

When fungi infect the skin it is one thing, but when fungi enter the body after a cut or scrape, it now has access far beyond our skin. A skin fungal infection is known as a *local mycosis*, whereas once fungus gains access to the inside of the body via a break in the skin, unless our immune system defeats it, it is known as a *systemic mycosis*. These are referred to throughout this book.

There are many practitioners who would assert that if you repeatedly have a fungal infection on your skin, you likely have fungal overgrowth inside your body, too, most likely in the gut. Chronic topical fungal problems, in other words, could be an outward sign of internal fungal problems. This is key when considering the influence of fungi and their mycotoxins on skin health. This obviously also leads us to ask whether fungi could cause skin problems deeper than the obvious skin infections. Let's take a closer look at some of the more subtle problems that occur with the skin.

Age-Related Skin Problems

No one escapes the ravages of time, and there is likely no clearer evidence of a person's age than their skin. Age-related skin damage, while a natural part of getting older, is evidenced by wrinkles, facial movement lines, dry and itching skin, loose skin (particularly in the face), bruising easily and age spots. All of these symptoms are caused by a variety of factors, including gravity, daily facial and skin movements, stress and loss of fatty tissue between the skin and muscle.

The number one contributor to age-related skin degeneration, we are told, is the sun. It is true that sunlight exposure creates free radicals in the skin that breakdown connective tissue, or collagen, but I don't believe that the sun is God's mistaken way of deteriorating your skin. The advice most of us have heard when it comes to preserving skin health is to stay out of the sun or use sunscreen when you are out in the sun.

Have you ever stopped to question that advice? We know moderate sunlight exposure can actually be good for your skin and overall health. To some, it seems like something as natural as the sun catches far too much blame for destroying our skin than it deserves. We cannot escape the sun, and we would not live even if we could. We need the sun! Just as you would not light a match and hold on to it until it burns your fingers, you also know that excessive exposure to the suns rays will burn your skin. Don't do it, as eventually free radical damage will be obvious on your skin.

Fungi and Free Radical Damage

We are told that most skin damage occurs because of free radicals. How in the world are we exposed to those? Keep reading! Consider, to some extent that damage is damage. Whether you wrap your car around a tree, a telephone pole or a light post, the damage will look the same. Damage to your skin is no different. It may look the same, whether the cause is harsh chemicals in lotions, free radicals or something else we have not considered. This book is filled with "things we have not considered," so let's take that less traveled road. If we do not know what that "something" we have not considered is, we cannot know for sure if we are making the right calls when we avoid harsh chemicals and too much sunlight. Missing the cause enables medical researchers to recommend and create products for greater defenses against the causes that we know. But what if there are other causes of free radical damage that actually create more skin damage? What else could cause free radical damage to our skin?

Cut an apple in half; place one half in the refrigerator, leave the other half on the counter, and go to work. Eight hours later, the half left on the counter has aged terribly and looks as though it has rusted, while the half in the refrigerator is still white and looks like it was just cut. Why is that?

We are told that free radical damage, or oxidation, caused the apple left on the counter to break down and age so quickly. Experts tell us that the exposed apple just lost electrons; that is all. Indirectly, this may be the case, but how did healthy food cells lose electrons? If we could only figure this out, perhaps we would better understand what caused your skin diagnosis as it relates to free radical damage or oxidation.

What causes free radical damage or oxidation to begin with? Free radical damage, they say, imparts advanced aging onto our skin, so it is relevant to this chapter. Let's study this more carefully.

Free radical cells are cells with unpaired electrons; normal cells have a positive (+) and a negative (-) charge, but free radical cells do not. Why? What changed or unpaired their charge? The same is true of oxidation, a process in which a charge (electron) is lost. So technically, free radical damage and oxidation are identical.

Like many things in science, our brightest and best tend to shrug their shoulders and say, "Gosh, oxidation is a huge problem. I wish we knew how it occurred!" Think about cancer or diabetes or your miserable skin disease, and doctors make that exact statement. So, we just have free radical damage and oxidation of our cells, and we blame oxygen or the sun for it. The common answer to our skin problems seems to be just slather some white chemical concoction on your skin when you are outside, and you'll be fine! That answer requires an entire chapter of its own, so let's not go there. You did not buy this book to study medical controversies; you bought it because you have skin problems!

There is little oxygen in the refrigerator where I stored the other half of the apple, yet plenty in the kitchen. So, we tend to reason that the refrigerator-stored apple was exposed to less oxygen, while the half of the apple on the counter was exposed to a lot of oxygen. Problem solved and case closed! It was obviously the oxygen that caused unpaired electrons in the apple! Are we guilty of being a bit naive? A few years ago, a research paper was published that helped me better understand why the apple left on my kitchen counter rusted so quickly. We are told that the oxygen in my kitchen caused the rusting on the apple, but since fungus is everywhere, I began to think that *it is not oxygen that caused the apple to rust, rather the fungi in the oxygen*. Both oxygen and fungi are ubiquitous—they are everywhere, but only fungi cause rust.

Researchers blame the sun and oxygen for our skin problems, and medical schools teach that; dermatologists "educate" the patients of that fact! Why aren't they taught that it isn't the oxygen that causes free radical damage? It's fungus! The air we breathe has both oxygen and fungus in it. Fungus is fully capable of breaking down exposed apple cells and can even negatively impact their electron charges. The same is true of your skin. Exposure to oxygen (innocent), and therefore to fungus (guilty), may be playing a large role in your skin problem(s). You can know in a very short period of time as you will learn.

The fungus *Aspergillus* makes a poisonous mycotoxin called aflatoxin. Aflatoxin causes human liver cancer, so it is extremely toxic. The research paper I mentioned stated that aflatoxin interacts with various biochemical processes inside our bodies that impact the electron transport chain involved in supplying our cells with energy. That process continues and eventually leads to breakage of our DNA. Think about it. If this fungal mycotoxin called aflatoxin is capable of causing human cancer, it mutates your human DNA. While researching this subject, I simply typed *mycotoxin induced oxidation* into a common search engine and about 90,000 articles appeared. In layman's terms, it is extremely important to know this, because many doctors don't know it. Mycotoxins are poisonous to human cells and can cause them to lose or un-pair their electrons. So, you are left with two distinct choices; live in your refrigerator, or clean your HVAC and ducting systems in your home, thereby minimizing your exposure to mold (fungal) mycotoxins. While our researchers are publishing articles on new procedures and drugs to make your skin more beautiful, perhaps this cleaning alone might quickly improve your skin, since HVAC systems are sometimes so filled with mold spores.

That, however, is not all; there are plenty of reasons to consider my-cotoxins. First and foremost, remember that their job is to break down cells for the next generation to use. We know they cause damage; that is what they were made to do. Remember that list from chapter two showing all the ways that mycotoxins can hurt us? I introduced you to the knowledge that they are poisonous to our DNA (genotoxic) cells (cytotoxic), and so forth. One item on the list is dermatotoxic, or poisonous to the skin. For all these reasons, it makes sense that damage caused by mycotoxins would appear to be free-radical dam-age. It is fungi that produce mycotoxins in order to break down their immediate environment into absorbable nutrients.

There is more published evidence that mycotoxins can cause skin problems. *Health Canal* reported in 2015 on a discovery presented by scientists from Brown University and the University of California–San Francisco. They demonstrated that an enzyme secreted by the fungus *Pseudogymnoascus destructans* is responsible for causing white-nose syndrome in bats, which has killed large swaths of bat populations. The enzyme, aptly dubbed *Destructin-1*, is responsible for destroying collagen in bats.

So, we have a mycotoxin—a poisonous fungal metabolite—destroy-ing collagen cells in bats. The natural question to follow is, if fungus can destroy collagen in bats, what is preventing it from causing col-lagen damage in humans? Bats and humans are both mammals and our collagen is the same kind of tissue. Might fungus play a role in—or even be responsible for—the damages leading to age-related skin problems? Know that there is far too much money in bringing products to the market that treat bad skin for researchers to try to figure out the role of mycotoxins in causing the skin damage, but I can tell you what I'd do. I'd use a computer search engine to find the ingredient listed on skin restoration or treatment products that are thought to promote youthfulness, then carefully list the ingredient name followed by the word *anti-fungal* in my search. If the ingredient contains anti-fungal properties, it may just work for you *because of that very reason*! The product developing scientists may never know, but now you do. Pure aloe vera plant gel is documented as having great anti-fungal properties, and this plant has helped so many skin sufferers. Now you know why.

Skin Problems: An Overview of the Most Often "Deeper Issue"

The process of aging, ingestion of chemicals, oxidation and sun damage are not the only concerns you have with your body's largest organ. There are a variety of problems that can plague the human skin. Let us take a look at some of them and the factors your doctor may tell you are thought to cause them.

Acne

Acne is characterized by the appearance of blackheads, whiteheads, cysts, nodules and pustules on the skin. It can appear on your face, back, chest, neck, shoulders, arms and buttocks. Acne is caused by dead skin cells collecting in pores along with skin oil, resulting in ripe conditions for the flourishing of certain bacteria. The bacteria and your body's reaction to it causes your skin to become red and inflamed, allowing for nodules and pustules to form.

Particularly during adolescence, nearly all of us become familiar with the occasional pimple and periodic breakouts of more than one pimple. Chronic acne, however, is the most common skin condition in the United States; an estimated 40-50 million people are suffering with acne at any time with a growing number of adults suffering from the condition. Women, it appears, are the most vulnerable. Dermatologists, however, remain unclear as to why the incidence of adult acne is on the rise.

If you go to a doctor to treat your acne, chances are you will be placed on strong rounds of antibiotics. Antibiotics may not always be effective, though, and acne often returns in many sufferers. It is important to note that acne is an immune-system reaction, and mycotoxins are known to negatively affect the human immune system.

Psoriasis

People who suffer from psoriasis experience thick, white, silvery and red patches of skin called plaques. Skin cells growing too quickly cause this plaque. Psoriasis is a chronic condition that primarily affects adults. It is thought to be caused by an over reactive immune system, but environmental conditions can cause psoriasis flare-ups for some people.

Infections, stress, anxiety and certain medicines are known to make psoriasis worse. Interestingly, it is known that drinking alcohol, smoking and certain foods can causes psoriasis flares. Given that alcohol (itself a mycotoxin), cigarette smoke (often contaminated with mycotoxins) and certain segments of our food supply are often contaminated with mycotoxins, it would make sense to at least consider fungi and mycotoxins as contributing to psoriatic flare-ups, especially given its link to the immune system.

Eczema

The term eczema can describe a number of conditions in which the skin becomes dry and/or irritated. It is more common in infants and children. Generally speaking, eczema affects the face, scalp, wrists, hands, back of the knees and feet. Eczema appears as a rash and is often very itchy. Eczema can produce an oozing and crusting condition, particularly in infants.

The exact cause of eczema is unknown, but it is thought to be associated with an overactive immune system response. One thing that is known about eczema is that fungal conditions can cause this particular problem; people with allergies and asthma are at a greater risk of developing eczema. This is particularly interesting as it relates to the fungus link theory. There are very strong links between fungus and the incidence of asthma and allergies. If fungus can cause and/or exacerbate allergies, and if those conditions are thought to increase the risk of eczema, you can see how a strong link exists between the presence of fungi and the incidence of eczema.

Fungus and Your Skin Problems

We know that fungal infections of the skin are common. In *Principles and Practices of Clinical Mycology*, Dr. Matsumoto writes, "The dermatophytoses are amongst the most common diseases of humans."

(Dermatophytoses is the clinical term for fungal diseases of the skin.) The first line of chapter two in *Fungous Diseases* states that, "Mycotic infections of the skin are exceedingly common occurrences…" Throughout the chapter, Dr. Jacobson goes on to describe an array of fungal infections of the skin. Often, you will find the descriptions of the manifestations of fungal infections as plaques, pustular or scaling.

This is not to say conditions such as psoriasis or eczema or acne are purely fungal problems necessarily, but it is interesting that documented in the medical literature are descriptions of fungal problems that seem closely aligned with descriptions of diseases now known as acne, eczema and psoriasis. In reviewing Dr. Weakley's patient's charts with him 30 years ago, it was quite common to see his diagnosis, followed immediately by the two words, *unknown etiology*, meaning of unknown cause. Once he witnessed the fungus link to their skin problems, he could proudly erase those words. The diagnoses varied, but so often the cause did not.

Recall that many practitioners contend that if you have a chronic yeast infection anywhere on your body, you very likely have an internal yeast problem, which is likely in the gut as well. If you are struggling with a skin condition, such as acne or psoriasis, it may be useful to ask yourself a few questions. Is your diet rich in grains, corn, alcohol or other foods potentially contaminated with mycotoxins? Have you recently been on antibiotics? Have you at any time taken multiple rounds of antibiotics? Most antibiotics are mycotoxins that are derived from fungi. These antibiotics can aid in fueling a fungal infection in your gut. Antibiotics kill all bacteria, good and bad. Your gut's health depends on maintaining a balance between good bacteria and the *Candida* yeast that you were born with. Antibiotics upset this balance with a biological double whammy: They kill good bacteria that are supposed to be there, and they encourage yeast that shared space with this good bacteria to become more aggressive. When disease-causing fungi overgrow in your gut, they compromise your skin from the inside out, meaning that the eczema, psoriasis and possibly even acne on your skin is coming out from underneath.

We also cannot forget what you may be sick of hearing me say by now. Fungus is everywhere. Our skin is in contact with the air, water and everything we touch. Put these details together, and it is almost impossible to imagine that fungus is not a factor in many diseases, including skin disease.

Skin Health Without Products

Skin products of all kinds represent a billion-dollar industry. If fungi are at the root of many skin problems, using skin care products may be less necessary than we are led to believe. It makes good sense, then, that a diet designed to limit exposure to mycotoxins while starving any sort of disease-causing fungi would aid both in clearing up skin problems and supporting healthy skin. As the gut tissue goes, so goes the skin. If certain skin products are currently helping you, try finding out why by searching the anti-fungal link to them.

It sounds crazy to suggest that nature is insufficient to help us have healthy skin and that we have just been waiting around for all these centuries for humans to discover new products to treat our skin that can be quickly patented so profits can be made. The advice you will get in a dermatologist's office likely will not include a simple dietary test that may help pinpoint the root cause of your skin problems. However, if after three to six weeks on the Kaufmann Diet your skin appears clear, vibrant and youthful, you may wish to continue this diet for extended periods. As Dr. Weakley did long ago, you may just discover what has eluded you for decades.

Solutions for Skin Problems

What Can I Do If I Have a Rash or Other Skin Problems?

Earlier I promised I would tell you about the program we used with Dr. David Weakley's patients. I need to point out that this was decades ago, and at that time we did not know everything that we have explored in this book. We only suspected that fungus was at the root of almost everything unknown; we did not have the proof that is more plentiful today if you know where to find it. When he had an unknown cause, he put patients on two prescription anti-fungal drugs called Diflucan and Nystatin and a specialized diet that literally starved fungus from their bodies. This diet is essential and will be expounded upon in this book.

First, I would ask each patient if they had been on many rounds of antibiotics, if they drank excessively or how often they ate corn, wheat and peanuts; these three products can expose a person to fungal mycotoxins. Additionally, I would inquire about the age of their house, if it had ever leaked or flooded and how long they had lived in it. Most importantly, I asked them to detail their skin problems for me with heavy emphasis on when the condition began. Usually skin problems, if they have a fungal cause, can be traced back to the time that they were exposed heavily to fungal mycotoxins, and each of these questions assisted me in doing that. At the end of this book, I have included a *Spore Score* test to help you better understand how you may be exposed to fungus. While certainly not conclusive, it does help to gather the data needed to know if fungus may be causing your skin problem.

Whereas most doctors prescribe drugs to treat the cause of a disease, we did not have a cause for these patients. What we had was bad skin, tears and notes from 6 other doctors' offices, each trying to help with guess work. It amazed me how many drugs and therapies some of his patients had unsuccessfully used! The purpose for the Diflucan and Nystatin was experimental. We knew that they were safe and that we would only keep the patients on them for a few weeks before reaching our goal of identifying or ruling out fungus as the cause. The Internet was brand new then, and some patients were concerned about taking the two drugs. We had never experienced any bad reactions from them, but we knew that Diflucan was potentially toxic to the liver. The other drug, Nystatin, had no side effects. Diflucan assisted in cleansing the bloodstream and internal organs of fungus, whereas Nystatin treated the bowel. In other words, Diflucan carried the trash to the backdoor, and Nystatin took it to the waste cans. We used psyllium hulls (which is a natural health food store product) to bind these mycotoxins in the colon and assure their removal. Psyllium aids in regularity, which is a problem that seems to plague many skin sufferers. 30 years ago, I thought these anti-fungal drugs were the only way to go. Truly, at the time, they represented a breakthrough as a logical approach that worked, but today I have learned much more. Dr. Weakley would often sit down with me at the end of a busy day with various patient charts, and we would go over them together. He was truly amazed at the results he was witnessing with anti-fungal drugs and a changed diet.

A Better Way

Now that we know fungus is the root cause of so many diseases, do we need pharmaceuticals to help us confirm it? During the past 3 decades I have studied and learned so much. If I had cancer, or coronary artery disease, or diabetes or a serious neurological disease, I would still opt for these two drugs in combination with The Kaufmann Diet for a few weeks. However, because these skin problems are rarely life-threatening for most people, making some precise changes in their diet and lifestyle can enable them to accomplish the same goal without drugs.

Let's look, then, at the specialized diet I used with Dr. Weakley's patients all those years ago. It has long been my belief that many skin problems exist because the bowels are not working correctly, quite often because a nasty fungal infection exists within the intestines. For that reason, we recommended that patients take health store psyllium fiber for a few weeks to get the bowels moving. This is in addition to eliminating the foods that fungi thrive on. The diet has never been a static diet, since I continue to learn. For example, 30 years ago, I used to think that quinoa and amaranth were grains, but I have since learned that they are seeds and therefore perfectly OK to eat while on The Kaufmann Diet.

I cannot say enough about how important it is to make big changes when you are dealing with skin problems. Your gut will not heal itself with incremental changes, and some of you will suffer far longer than you need to.

Foods to Avoid

Many of your favorites will be on this list. Sugar, corn, potatoes, most grains and any foods containing them are at the top of the list of foods to avoid. Sugar, foods high in sugar and starches all feed fungi, particularly in your gut. Other foods high in fungus and mycotoxins include peanuts, mushrooms, pistachios and sometimes, albeit rarely, even coffee.

Get a calendar with boxes for each date, and put an X in each day you go without the things that are hardest to give up. Challenge yourself to see how many days in a row you can go without them. Since this is not a life-threatening disease and you have time, if you miss a day, don't kick yourself. Start a new streak.

Your skin and perhaps even your life truly does depend on how well you do these things. It is practically true that eating and drinking mycotoxin-contaminated food is like eating and drinking tiny doses of poison on a regular basis.

Foods to Include

Grass-fed beef, buffalo, or lamb, wild-caught fish and free-range, flaxseed-fed chicken are all high in Omega-3 fatty acids. Eggs are also a great source of protein. There are brands and varieties of Omega-3 eggs in most grocery stores and these are even better for you. If you like salads, you are in luck. Green leafy vegetables, cruciferous vegetables and green vegetables are among the best. Fruits are high in fiber, but they are also high in sugar, so eat the ones detailed in the Kaufmann Diet (at the end of the book) and keep them in moderation.

Supplements

There are hundreds of options for anti-fungal supplements in every health food store, although they will not be labeled as anti-fungal supplements. These include amino acids, omega fatty acids, caprylic acid, vitamin C, D3 and resveratrol to name a very few. I also recommend taking a daily probiotic before bed, which is a great way to restore your gut balance as you make efforts to starve fungus.

CHAPTER 8

I Don't Have a Fungal Problem! I'm Going Through Menopause!

During my almost 5 decades in the healthcare world, I have seen so many scientific advancements. Some have been lifesaving, and some don't seem to me to be advancements at all. Childbirth and menopause, in my humbled male opinion, are not diseases, yet they certainly generate a lot of doctor office visits and prescriptions. (Don't get me wrong; it is always a good idea to visit a doctor when concerns abound for your safety or that of an unborn child.) The dictionary defines menopause as the period of permanent cessation of menstruation, usually occurring between the ages of 45 and 55. I'm left to wonder what a doctor can do for a normal physiological event in your life, like menopause. After all, what did he do for your puberty?

Since many of us think of our doctors' role as more of a symptom eraser than as a healthcare facilitator, we tend to view anything they treat as a problem. Rather than understanding that menopause happens to women as a natural "change of life" evolution, some doctors unfortunately tend to talk about menopause as though it were an illness, and the pharmaceutical industry is called on to solve it. They run commercials for their drugs on TV and the Internet which only deepens the misunderstanding among the public. If you are currently going through menopause, you might think you have a disease. I now feel that we are witnessing the age of medical over-diagnosis and over-treatment. Over treatment has its costs, and I believe it tends to rob many women of the joy of entering a new season in life. I know that is easy for any male to say, but do you agree that this change is a natural part of the aging process? If so, know that while I can't assist you in stopping menopause, I may be able to assist in calming the symptoms of menopause. Along with the dietary changes recommended in this book, I have long recommended a visit to a naturopathic doctor (ND) for recommendations on bio-identical hormone replacement and perhaps some natural anti-fungal supplements. Now, let's learn more about menopause.

Menopause is anything but a joyful time for many women. For some, menopause comes with more pain than joy and for others, there is no joy in it at all. There are many reasons why it may be a time of grief. Your childbearing years are ending. Your hormones are changing. Your body is changing in other, more visible ways. You are being faced with your own mortality. You feel like you are losing your final grip on your youth, and with it, your worth.

As a rapidly aging man, I am here to tell you that your worth is not at all dependent on your youth! At my ripe old age, here I am authoring another book, this time on the relationship that certain germs may have to menopause. The many menopausal women who sought my counsel throughout my career taught me well. I'm hoping that what I learned from them will pay dividends to you in this chapter.

Having caring people around treating you like you have a disease certainly does not help when going through menopause. If you have ever been pregnant, you have seen this before. Pregnancy is one of the most natural and beautiful things your body could ever experience. Some say that your body was made for pregnancy. Yet, because things can and do go wrong, doctors get involved to try to prevent them, and soon the entire process became a medical process instead of a natural one. Again, do not get me wrong. Having access to medical aid is a good thing. Trust me, if men birthed children, every baseball and football stadium in America would have birthing centers complete with 5 doctors, 12 anesthesiologists and 2 bartenders.

Every Woman's Path

Not all women experience pregnancy. However, all women will at some point experience the changes in body chemistry known as menopause. Menopause is a natural part of aging. The average age for a woman to experience menopause is 51. Menopause is caused by a natural decline in ovary function, resulting in the lowering of estrogen and other hormones. Menopause marks the permanent end of fertility in a woman; it also marks the end of menstruation. Menopause is considered confirmed when a woman has missed her periods for 12 consecutive months in the absence of other obvious causes.

While menopause is a natural part of aging and certainly not a disease, there are symptoms associated with menopause that most women are familiar with. These include irregular periods, vaginal dryness, hot flashes, night sweats, sleep problems, mood changes, weight gain, thinning hair, dry skin and loss of breast fullness. While the symptoms of menopause are not life threatening, they can be the source of discomfort for many women, and while going through menopause, these symptoms can interfere with the quality of a woman's life.

Preserving your quality of life is what got doctors into the menopause treatment business in the first place. To that end, your doctor may prescribe a variety of treatments. One benefit of modern medicine is that for every malady, there is often something your doctor can (and usually will) prescribe. This in itself can be a good thing, but when we start to look at what the associated risks of treatments are, we sometimes find that the benefits of treatments are far outweighed by the associated risks. Remember, almost all pharmaceutical medications have side effects, and they can often be worse than the symptoms they are treating. Each of you must decide for yourself if the recommended treatment is worth the risk that you are willing to take; this applies not only to menopause but blood pressure, cholesterol levels and even elective surgery. You must continuously educate yourself throughout your path in life.

I cannot tell you the number of healthy women who used to contact me after leaving their OB-GYN's office with prescriptions in hand.

"She said everything is fine, but she handed me two prescriptions to begin taking!"

Why?

"She said that all women benefit from taking hormone replacement therapy, because it lowers their breast cancer and heart disease risks."

Wow, I used to think to myself, what a boon for the pharmaceutical industry! Could doctors be correct in stating that the prophylactic use of estrogen and progestin prevented breast cancer and heart disease?

Of course, the study (Woman's Health Initiative) used to determine if our doctors were correct was halted unexpectedly in 2002 when just the opposite was confirmed long before the study was to end. As it turned out, these two prescription drugs actually *increased* the risk of breast cancer and heart disease. We must all become prudent medical consumers. But why were these hormones handed out like candy in OB-GYN offices for 50 years before this important study was begun? For the exact reason antibiotics are handed out in pediatric offices like candy today. I believe it was to usher in a new way of convincing doctors to prescribe medications.

As the WHI study was halted, no one can deny that much was learned by drug companies. HRTs had set the pharmaceutical stage for them to better understand our doctors' willingness to prescribe drugs to well patients. When the scientific whistle was blown for HRT drugs, drug company salespeople simply introduced physicians to statin drugs to be taken…by well people. Today, many millions of Americans are taking prophylactic statin drugs in hopes of preventing heart attacks. Recall that HRTs were dispensed to save woman's lives. This same mentality is being used to sell statin drugs today. Statins' day will come, I am certain, and these too will be identified as knowingly problematic from the beginning. Until that time, it is not the pharmaceutical companies' or your doctors' job to know the side effects that you may experience or the inherent dangers of statin drugs or any other drug that you may take. That is your job, since you will be the one swallowing them! Always keep this fact in the back of your mind when being handed a prescription; when I was born, 4 out of 5 doctors smoked

Camel cigarettes! This was as heavily promoted as drugs are today. Please be careful and judicious, because they used to smoke and now they prescribe drugs. In addition to their other duties, it's just what they do.

Now, let's learn more about HRT and this Woman's Health Initiative study.

Treating Menopause: Risk vs. Reward

If you walk into your doctor's office seeking relief from the symptoms of menopause, there are a variety of ways he or she may treat your symptoms. It largely depends on the symptoms and their severity. Understandably, many women seek their doctor's help for hot flashes, night sweats and complications that make sex difficult or less enjoyable such as vaginal dryness. Generally, to meet these needs, your doctor will prescribe some type of hormone replacement therapy, the thinking being that nature needs help when your body stops producing hormones at the levels it once did.

Hormone replacement therapy generally involves prescribing estrogen, and in cases where a woman has not had her uterus removed by partial hysterectomy, progestin will be added to the prescription. In cases of vaginal dryness, vaginal estrogen is often prescribed as well. Like many drugs, hormone replacement therapy, or HRT, was hailed as a miracle cure for menopause when it was released so long ago, and following its introduction, HRT was routinely prescribed to women entering the years of menopause. Women were told they would maintain youthful appearance, feel more energy, have heightened libido and be free of the symptoms that plagued their mothers through menopause. Little research was needed, as HRT drugs were simply handed out like candy in any OB-GYN's office. This became common practice before there was enough time to know what the long-term effects could possibly be. Although the long-term darker side of these "therapies" remained to be seen, they are now well published.

In 2002, The Women's Health Initiative (WHI) released a study implicating hormone replacement therapy in the increased risk of stroke, heart attack, blood clots and breast cancer. Years of wantonly prescribing hormones to women had caused untold misery and even death. This obviously caused a substantial drop in the number of prescriptions and number of women receiving hormone replacement therapy.

Unfortunately, this is a trend often seen in medicine: A blockbuster drug is introduced and hailed as a silver bullet. The companies releasing the drug rake in astronomically high profits. Thereafter, we learn the drug's side effects were more profound than those revealed by the clinical trials. Oops! This boom/bust cycle remains lucrative for the companies selling drugs. They can make enough on the front end to pay out millions in settlements on the back end and still have enormous profits. This may be great for their bottom line, but what about the rest of the general public whose lives and families are affected?

Astoundingly, many of these drugs are not even removed from the market. Instead, they are simply prescribed with a black box warning. This warning is somehow supposed to be a deterrent, but what patient will be warned off of a drug when their doctor has prescribed it to them? How many of us just take what the doctor prescribes, because we trust that the doctor knows best? Then, how many doctors prescribe those drugs, because the pharmaceutical sales rep told them the black box warning is just red tape and the drug is safe? We don't know the answer to the many questions that surround black box warnings. This scenario highlights much of the confusion in modern medicine at best, but perhaps underscores what might just be the nefarious, cynical attitude of Big Pharma.

Years from now, if your daughters are experiencing the symptoms of menopause, estrogen replacement is likely the first thing their doctor will suggest to treat their symptoms. While it is understandable for people to seek relief from symptoms, it makes me wonder if there is something more deeply embedded in our collective psyche that is causing women to choose therapies that run the risk of causing life-threatening conditions. Do you ever feel like that?

Big Business: Selling Youth

An accountant friend of mine has a sign nicely framed behind his desk. It reads, "A man spends his first 45 years of his life gaining his wealth and the next 45 years buying back his health."

So it is today. Yes, we work hard to gain our wealth, but at what cost? We live in a time and culture that places an unprecedented value on youth which is often gone at age 45. This cultural obsession with anti-aging drives a booming business that aims to sell people back their health and their youth. Look no further than the boom in businesses such as cosmetic surgery, weight loss clinics and botox clinics.

We should be clear here: It is a noble goal to maintain one's health, fitness and vibrance throughout all stages of life, but how are these categorized as "health fixes?" Health is a goal we ourselves wish to promote. However, when people regularly go under the knife or inject botulism toxin into their body, I have got to wonder about how healthy our obsession is with staying young. Certainly there are better ways of maintaining both health and youth. As I have said before, our bodies were simply not made to be opened and closed like a ziplock bag.

Hormone replacement therapy, as you might remember, was hailed as a fountain of youth for women. At a time in history when youth is so highly prized, hormone therapy might as well be the gold standard. While the Women's Health Initiative might have caused a decline in the number of hormone replacement therapies prescribed, hormones have likely never been so en vogue—and not just for women. Men are routinely encouraged to receive hormone therapy more than ever before as well.

The risks of hormone replacement therapy have been well documented, yet it is still the most common way women are told to deal with menopause in America. While these risks are known—and more will likely continue to reveal themselves—there remains another risk associated with hormones that may often be overlooked.

The Relationship Between Fungus and Hormones

Were you starting to wonder if I had forgotten to talk about the link to fungus? Hormones and fungi have a unique relationship. We have discussed how fungal poisons called mycotoxins can interfere with normal hormone function. The mycotoxin, zearalenone is known to cause hormonal problems in both animals and humans. *Fusarium* fungal species make this poisonous mycotoxin, and it is commonly known to those who study fungal poisons that *fusarium* commonly contaminates cereal grains. Yes, there was a simpler time in America when this information was unknown. Yet our mothers did have menopausal symptoms, and perhaps by better understanding endocrine disrupters like zearalenone, you can begin to see how they might play an important role in causing the symptoms that menopause brings for so many women.

What this means is, if you eat a diet rich in grains and meat—the Standard American Diet (SAD) that the majority of we Americans consume every day—there is a chance you are being exposed regularly to measurable amounts of mycotoxins including zearalenone and *fusarium* fungi (mold). If this is the case, and if you are experiencing symptoms related to hormone disruption, mycotoxins could be the root cause of your problems. If they are not the root cause, they may most certainly be making the problems worse. Regardless, your doctor would likely never implicate your diet, much less fungal contaminants or disease-causing fungi as the cause of hormone-related issues. This is simply not taught in medical schools.

We have seen examples of what fungi and their mycotoxins can do to hormones, but what can hormones do to fungi? Certain disease-causing species of fungi, such as *Candida*, are known to thrive in the presence of estrogen. The risk of vaginal yeast infections is known to increase in the presence of high-estrogen contraceptive therapy. Estrogen also increases the adherence of yeasts to vaginal skin cells. We also know that yeast infections are more common in women with elevated estrogen levels including women who are pregnant. It is even well documented that women who are on estrogen therapy are at risk for getting yeast infections. It is becoming very nearly impossible to deny these connections!

Knowing these things raises a logical question: Are women who are prescribed estrogen therapy at a greater risk of developing not just a superficial vaginal yeast infection but a systemic fungal infection with broader implications?

The side effects associated with estrogen therapy may, themselves, be clues to the associated fungal problems estrogen replacement therapies put you at risk for. There is also an established link between hormone therapy and the risk of breast cancer as we will see in a later chapter. While we have known of the cancer fungus/link for many years, it is a new idea to mainstream medicine. Perhaps time will reveal what the real cause of many breast cancers is and what the subsequent risks of estrogen therapy are. But HRT may not be fully responsible for the high rate of breast cancer in American women. As you may know, the diagnosis of estrogen-receptor-positive breast cancer rates have skyrocketed in America today, and according to the American Cancer Society, 2 out of 3 breast cancers diagnosed today are ER+. What this means to you and me is cancer cells may be receiving signals from estrogen, or estrogen mimickers, that promote their growth. What is the fungus-breast cancer link? Given that these poisonous fungal mycotoxins can be both carcinogenic and estrogenic (mimic a woman's own estrogen), this subject needs to be tackled in this book and it will be. Keep reading!

Going Through Menopause Naturally

I know what you must be thinking; if I do not want to subject my body to the ravages of hormone replacement therapy, what can I do to get through these hot flashes?! I understand. Let me invite you to make some radical changes in your diet and the way you live. I personally know women who have followed my Kaufmann Lifestyle and Diet and have not experienced any of the symptoms of menopause. Are they exceptions to the rule, and is it possible that their experience can be yours? Many of you reading this book are currently going through menopause and might feel that making dietary changes may be too late now. It may not be, as many women who begin the Kaufmann Diet have reported to me that their symptoms began diminishing within a week of starting the diet that is meant to starve parasitic yeasts and fungi. What have you to lose by adopting this lifestyle for a month or two and determining for yourself if your menopausal symptoms might be linked to one or more of the commonly consumed mycotoxins in our diet?

My friend, Dr. Christine Salter, once told me personally, "The issue is that most women are prescribed estrogen without the balance of bio-identical progesterone." What this means is that the estrogen you get in hormone replacement therapy is a chemical derivative (from pregnant mare urine, no less!) instead of a hormone produced by your body. This is something your doctor might be dismissive about, but given the list of side effects related to estrogen therapy, it seems like a good idea to ask questions about bio-identical hormone replacement in lieu of what many doctors prescribe.

CHAPTER 9

I Don't Have a Fungal Problem! I Have Fibromyalgia and Fatigue!

This will be a long chapter for two reasons; most people who suffer from fibromyalgia and chronic fatigue are females. Additionally, so many women have requested that I write on fibromyalgia and chronic fatigue as they might relate to fungus. The subject is deep and a bit intense, but we will go where other books have not gone. At the end of this chapter lies hope. I've added a powerful virtual office visit (wait until you read this!) with a female physician friend of mine who understands fungus as well as anyone. I truly believe that this information will be as life changing for many of you as it was for so many patients in the doctors' offices where I worked in the past. Remember, we are all unique thumbprints when it comes to our health. Find your course of action—your thumbprint—in this chapter, and I believe so many questions will be answered for you!

The year was 1988. I was working in Texas with two dermatologists and a general practitioner who was also board certified in dermatology. The doctor that signed our 5-year agreement had travelled to Los Angeles and knew of my ability to help people, many of whom had lost hope. I had developed an anti-fungal protocol by using anti-fungal drugs (if the doctor would prescribe them), supplements and a diet that is today called The Kaufmann Diet. After witnessing the results first hand, he made me an offer to relocate my family to Texas for 5 years. I did. That was 31 years ago.

One of the best parts of working with dermatologists is interviewing their patients. As you will read at the end of this chapter, rarely does a patient have a skin condition without having many other symptoms. It was common for patients to tell the staff that they had to see the doctor quickly, because they had taken the afternoon off work and had three or four more doctor visits for other complaints. You see, dermatologists, while medical doctors, don't see patients that are depressed, or that have stomach complaints or eye problems. That is a job for several other doctors...all called "specialists."

Yes, these patients had psoriasis and eczema and strange skin diseases like granuloma annulare, but the great majority also had fibromyalgia, stomach problems, fatigue and depression. As I would interview those patients that the doctors felt they had failed, I found this pattern to exist over and over again. I recall thinking that skin diseases might be systemic problems not merely affecting just the patients' skin.

I do not recall the first patient that complained of whole body muscle pain, but by 1989, the doctors probably had 10 of these systemic pain patients, all complaining of the same types of symptoms, including horrible pain and stiffness, fatigue, anxiety, fading memory and (of course) stomach problems.

I approached the doctors and requested that they consider the same anti-fungal program I had initiated that was so successful for their skin disease patients. The senior doctor was concerned as to whether or not this muscle pain was even a disease. After examining the patients, he finally told me that he became a doctor to help people, and although perhaps a long shot, he thought my program had the potential to help them. For his skin patients that had failed traditional therapy and now for this new group of systemic pain patients, he routinely prescribed two anti-fungal drugs (Diflucan and Nystatin), and I educated each of their patients on the diet and supplements that I recommended.

The doctors would follow up with these new systemic pain patients at 14 days and then again at 30 days. For some, the anti-fungal approach was lifesaving—literally as one patient had become suicidal after suffering for over a year. Two weeks is rarely enough to reverse or cure a systemic yeast/fungal condition, but the early results lent hope to these patients who had no hope before. Within a few months, one patient had invited me to a local medical school in Ft. Worth, Texas, to give a lecture to a group of doctors on the results she had gotten using anti-fungal medications and a changed diet with her fibromyalgia. Even the doctors were surprised as many had never even seen a systemic pain patient. In essence, they now had a viable treatment option before they even had a disease. Within a few years, however, every physician knew what fibromyalgia was.

It was not until 1990 that this strange illness was even classified as fibromyalgia. It has since been categorized as an autoimmune disorder, meaning that the disease, its cause and treatment options remain largely unknown. Once again, these fibromyalgia patients are relegated to a life of doctor visits, medications and a lifetime of a disease that progresses without an end in sight. In their doctors' defense, since they did not learn of systemic fungal diseases in their medical training, such an approach is entirely logical.

A Dual Disease for Many

Fibromyalgia affects about 5-6% of the American population and, as I mentioned, affects far more women than men. About 70% of those who have fibromyalgia also have another disease, called chronic fatigue syndrome, or CFS. This makes life nearly unbearable for most as the waking hours are spent exhausted and in severe pain.

What Causes Fibromyalgia and CFS?

I had this same question in 1988 and saw the concerns that the doctors I worked with had when I approached them about trying the anti-fungal program in their clinic for these patients. Far too often, patients are examined, tests are ordered, blood is drawn and the patient is scheduled to come back in a week or so when the lab results come in. Another week of misery is exactly what these patients do not need, yet they hang on to hope that perhaps this doctor will find what the previous doctors did not. To make matters worse for them, once the lab work comes in, it reveals very little with regard to their health problems. There isn't a blood test that screams, "She has fibromyalgia!" We rely on the use of old tests for new diseases.

I want you to really think for a moment; recall that I requested the doctors to prescribe two anti-fungal drugs for fibromyalgia patients. I then taught them how to follow my diet, a diet that starves fungus. If fibromyalgia were not a fungal disorder, these drug and diet experiments would have been for naught. None of them would have improved, and we would have all labeled this what many still do—a disease of unknown cause. Yet, several of their patients experienced dramatic symptom reversal within 30 days while on this program. What does that tell you? Perhaps not in all cases, but in some cases, mold (fungus) initiated the muscle pain and perhaps even the accompanying symptoms.

Are you one of the cases that would have improved in our clinic? If so, what might we have all concluded? Do you see where I am going with this? Symptoms and/or diseases never, ever respond favorably to an anti-fungal program unless they are fungal symptoms and/or diseases. Based on this, let me share with you what helped some of these patients so many years ago and then update you on what I have learned since then.

What We Recommended in 1989

If you suffer from either one or both of these illnesses, you do not need 10 more pages that list symptoms and recommended medical treatments. You have been down that road for many years without finding the answers. Rather, you need a program that offers hope, not only for symptom relief, but almost as important for the scientist in all of you, you need to understand what might have caused these years of misery.

Let us start with the cause. If within 30 days you find yourself feeling much better, then we are on the right track. The years have taught me, however, that most women want more than clinical improvement; they want answers! Know that the program you are about to embark upon does nothing more than starve and kill fungus. So if you respond well in a short period of time, logic might dictate that somewhere, somehow fungus was able to enter your body, and it started your misery.

At the end of this book, we provide you with what I will call a fungal exposure Spore Score test. Some of the questions that might apply to your illness have their roots in past or current fungal exposure. For example, as a child or even more recently, have you taken many rounds of antibiotics? Do you recall living in a home that leaked or smelled like mildew or mold? Do you crave pasta, bread, sugar or carbohydrates? At any time in your life have you worried about your alcohol consumption? The foods that seem to expose us the most to toxic, mycotoxin-containing molds are generally peanuts and corn of any type and all grains more broadly. If you were anything like me in my youth, then you lived on popcorn, corn on the cob, corn sweeteners and peanut butter. You see, each of these foods (and others) expose you to fungal mycotoxins that might be at the root of your fibromyalgia or CFS today.

Unfortunately, we tend to believe that once a round or two of antibiotics has been completed, you are good to go. Hundreds of scientific reports, however, now attest that antibiotics can cause damage many years from the time they are swallowed. Did you know that children who took many rounds of antibiotics tend to be overweight in their adult years? Antibiotics don't cause a 2 year old to become an obese 3 year old, but they can cause a child with many ear or throat infections a lifetime of hit and miss weight loss approaches. Perhaps one or more YES answers on the Spore Score test might assist you in better understanding the cause of your health problems today, so keep reading as I outline an old program that could be responsible for helping millions of people today.

In 1989, after listening to several of the doctors' patients tell me about their fibromyalgia, it was decided that the doctors would "rush to diagnosis" if you will, because there was deep concern as to what this miserable disease with no name might cause people to do—things that they would have otherwise had never done. When I tell you that sufferers were depressed, know that I have never seen depression this bad, and it concerned us all. In 2011, *Psychology Today* magazine, Mark Borigini, M.D., wrote a fabulous article entitled, *Fibromyalgia and Death*. In it, he quoted a Danish female fibromyalgia study. He stated, "Disturbingly, the suicide risk among fibromyalgia patients was ten times that of the general population." I cannot even imagine feeling that hopeless. Because of how hopeless these patients were, the doctors I worked with agreed to a 30-day trial of two prescription drugs. These were great, caring doctors! Besides, these two drugs were not fibromyalgia drugs; no such thing existed then. Rather, the approach was the trial of two anti-fungal drugs and a specialized anti-fungal diet.

Diflucan (200mg) was prescribed for 5 consecutive days, then one every other day for the next few weeks. Per their prescriptions, a total of 15 Diflucan pills were dispensed. Today, generic Diflucan is called fluconazole. Diflucan treats systemic or bloodstream and organ fungal conditions. It filters through the liver and can cause liver enzymes to elevate. It is known to be a potential liver toxin (hepatotoxic). For this reason, we would draw the patient's blood before prescribing it and again after 30 days or so and check these enzymes. (Just so you know, we never once witnessed an elevated liver enzyme in the years we were together).

Nystatin (500,000IU, hard tablets) was the second anti-fungal drug they prescribed; one after breakfast and one after dinner for 7 days, then 2 after breakfast and dinner, daily. They would prescribe a total of 180 tablets. It was always taken after a meal. Nystatin was developed in Albany, NY in 1950 by two female researchers, Dr. Hazen and Dr. Brown, hence the name, NY-State-In, or Nystatin! This is an extremely safe drug. It is prescribed to treat gut yeast infections, and I do not believe it is coincidental that Nystatin was approved by the FDA shortly after antibiotics came on the market. Once you begin to erase the good bacteria in the intestines, which antibiotics do, health rules all change for the worse. Antibiotics were lifesavers 75 years ago, and to a certain extent, they can still save lives today. But their more current, non-judicious use is unquestionably linked with far more than the antibiotic resistance they cause. This was predicted 40 years ago.

"It is ironic that this humbled fungus (penicillium), hailed as a benefactor of mankind, may by its very success prove to be a deciding factor in the decline of present day civilization."

– Dr. John Pitt, *The Genus Penicillium*, Academic Press, 1979

Both Diflucan and Nystatin can cause a die-off response, wherein the symptoms being treated may flare up a bit. If this occurs, the doctors would tell the patient to take half the dose for a few days, and this always seemed to help.

In Texas, we have a saying: *When you find a good horse, you ride it!* Once these very ill patients began to see relief, the doctors would again prescribe anti-fungal medications in hopes that more relief became evident. That all changed when the senior doctor unexpectedly died. I was devastated, and the medical partnership dissolved. I was on my own to find another way besides prescriptive anti-fungals that the doctors once supplied to help these then patients and now clients. Prescription medication was no longer available to me.

A few years later, I did work with another physician who I had met. Because of the nature of the health problems that I had witnessed, I felt it was best to work with a physician. It was thanks to this special physician that my business spread. Between his education in microbiology and his medical degree, he was eons beyond most physicians when it came to understanding fungus. As he examined patients in our clinic and began using the anti-fungal program, he quickly learned (as I had years ago) that fungus was a maligned and misunderstood field of science that had been totally overlooked. We were both so excited about the results we were seeing, and each week brought a new set of symptoms that neither of us would have ever linked to fungus unless we had seen recovery with our own eyes. More and more we witnessed the diet being the epicenter of the entire program. Did we really need anti-fungal drugs? He and I attended some courses on herbal nutrition and discovered that nature could supply anti-fungal relief without the concern of prescription drug-related injury. Mind you, we had never witnessed it, but the thought of reducing potential injury while accomplishing the exact end result excited us. Armed with new anti-fungal herbs and supplements and this diet, we began to work more closely with his patients' diets and less with a prescription pad. Retrospectively, I realize today that God placed this wonderful man in my life at a crucial time in my career. Although we only spent a few years together, they were the best years of my career and many, many people with symptoms and/or diseases of unknown cause were helped during these years. What was it about this diet that helped so many?

The Kaufmann Diet is based on the premise that when one has a fungal disease, one must eat what fungus does not! Fungi thrive on carbohydrates so for a period of time, if you have a fungal illness, you cannot. It really is that simple. More on this diet as the book progresses, but this diet is extremely important as it will relate to your discoveries about fibromyalgia and/or CFS.

The bowels were made to eliminate regularly. So many women with fibromyalgia were constipated, and I believe this actually worsens the disease. What good are medications or natural, plant-based anti-fungal supplements or even spinach when it sits in the gut and putrefies for 6 days? Through the years, I would learn that non-digestible forms of fiber aid in elimination. A green apple is a great form of digestible fiber, and in many cases, dietary fiber works to keep us regular. But as we become diseased, or even as we age, elimination sometimes becomes hampered. This is when non-digestible fiber can really help. Psyllium is such a fiber. Since it does not digest, what goes in eventually must come out. Fibers enhance peristalsis, so it aids in creating the urge to go to the bathroom. Most importantly, psyllium fiber binds these fungal mycotoxins; with enhanced peristalsis, old debris and disease-causing germs are moved out quickly.

I used to recommend psyllium fiber in a jar of water (shake very well) each night before going to bed. Usually, within a week, the bowels were responding favorably. With great food now going in and toxins being eliminated, symptoms would begin diminishing before too long, and health would begin to improve. I still remember seeing one of these deeply-pained individuals return to our office after 14 days and I recall thinking, "She looks totally different with a smile on her face!" Hope was upon us!

Recommendations for 2019
To this day, I have no problem requesting the two anti-fungal drugs, Diflucan and Nystatin, from your doctor, especially if you feel absolutely

hopeless. Just know that since very few doctors are armed with any understanding of the role of fungi or their poisonous mycotoxins in any disease process, your request may fall on deaf ears. So often, sufferers find themselves on their own. Do not be discouraged. In 2017, I authored this "physicians' educational" review that people could share with their doctors. Many physicians have prescribed anti-fungal drugs for their patients, and they have been helpful in their recovery process. This review is printable on my website, knowthecause.com.

Physician Educational: The Fungus Link and Prescribing Anti-fungal Medications

Dear Doctor,

Your patient has requested information on an anti-fungal protocol. I was a US Navy hospital corpsman, trained in emergency medicine and served in that capacity while attached to the 7th Marine Division in Vietnam. Upon returning home, I suffered from numerous symptoms. For years I attributed those to PTSD. Dr. Everett Hughes, with whom I was collaborating on research with at USC Medical School, suggested that, given my overseas deployment, perhaps my symptoms were due to a parasite. While studying parasitology, I discover that pathogenic fungi parasitize humans. Upon doing so, hosts often begin eating a carbohydrate-rich diet to satisfy the fungal parasites' cravings. Fungal secondary metabolites, mycotoxins, are commonly found in our American grain and peanuts supply and serve as a portal of entry. I developed a highly nutritional, yet carbohydrate-sparing diet in the 1970s that works wonderfully to "starve" fungi. Many have maintained this diet for over a decade, so it is quite safe. The diet is available in any of my 10 books, and I have developed my website (knowthecause.com) to teach the lay public about pathogenic fungi, their mycotoxins and systemic fungal infections. This diet is the genesis of the anti-fungal protocol.

Diet & Anti-fungal Drug Protocol

In August 2017, the CDC published that certain less-common fungi infections (Valley Fever and Candidemia) can cause serious illness and even death. Further, in addition to other factors, the CDC published that taking certain medications increased vulnerability to serious fungal infections. Fungal diseases, they wrote, are not diagnosed right away, because fungal symptoms can mimic other diseases. Finally, they apprised the general public to "think fungus" when their symptoms persist despite medical treatment. The CDC recommended that your patients talk to you about the possibility of a fungal infection. [1]

There are currently 610 papers on pubmed.gov highlighting the ability of fungal mycotoxins to induce genetic mutations. Mycotoxins are secondary metabolites produced by micro fungi that are capable of causing disease and death in humans and other animals. [2]

Exposure to mycotoxins is thought to be common. Our corn and groundnut supply is often contaminated with mycotoxins and is both plentiful and regularly consumed. Dietary exposure to Aspergillus mold is known as a hepatocellular carcinoma human risk factor. [3]

Parasitic fungi can thrive in a symbiotic relationship with their hosts, but they can also become obligates, in which case, they can feed at the expense of a host. At this point a patient can begin experiencing annoying or more severe symptoms. Unfortunately, diagnosing fungal disorders remains difficult and time consuming. For this reason, the short protocol outlined in this brief letter may assist you.

While many patients improve dramatically within 14 days on the anti-fungal diet alone, sometimes simply "starving" fungi is not always enough. For this reason, some of the physicians that I have consulted with also use short-term gut and systemic anti-fungal therapy simultaneously. The diet and anti-fungal drug protocol enabled the physician to quickly and safely rule out, or diagnose, a fungal condition. The anti-fungal drug protocol we have used for several years proved to be safe and efficacious, as we never once observed hepatotoxicity or any other adverse drug event while on this short-term anti-fungal drug protocol.

Nystatin 500,000 tabs #180
Sig: i po bid pc X 3d, thereafter ii po bid pc 1 re II

Fluconazole 200mg #14
Sig: 1/2 tab po qd X 2d, thereafter one po qod 1 re II

Itraconazole, or Sporanox, has recently made news in that it has been repurposed as a cancer chemotherapy drug [4].

In lieu of using Diflucan, some practitioners order Sporanox for their patients. Given the rise in both cancer cases and Aspergillus-induced fungal infections, this may be a good option for a short-term trial. Also, some practitioners rotate Sporanox and Diflucan every month or two due to the fact that each kills different fungi. For suspected Aspergillosis infections, 1-2 caps daily is recommended, as opposed to suspected Blastomycosis and Histoplasmosis infections, wherein 2 caps daily are recommended.

Sporanox 200mg #30
Sig: i-ii po pc qd. 1 re II

I have worked with many physicians in the past 4 decades and developed working models for the inclusion of anti-fungal programs in their practices. Most importantly, upon our follow up visits with each patient in 14 days, we observed results like we never had before. At that point, we terminated anti-fungal drugs in favor of anti-fungal supplements like Vitamin C, Vitamin D3, Caprylic Acid or Resveratrol, although some opted for routine liver tests and continuation on the anti-fungal drugs given their newfound relief. Patients loved the results and the fact that we enabled them more control *of their fungal symptoms. Many had finally achieved a diagnosis, an easy to follow anti-fungal protocol and hope. They referred many new patients to us.*

If I may be of further assistance to you, please don't hesitate to contact me, personally, M-F, at _____

Most Sincerely,
Doug A. Kaufmann

References
(1) Announcement: Fungal Diseases Awareness Week – August 14-18, 2017. MMWR morbidity and mortality Weekly, Rep 2017;66:837
(2) Clin. Microbiol. Rev. July 2003 vol. 16 no. 3 497-516
(3) J Gastrointestin Liver Dis. 2013 Sep;22(3):305-10
(4) Ecancermedicalscience. 2015; 9: 521

If your symptoms are less life threatening, not having access to anti-fungal drugs can actually be a blessing in disguise; I have always been a proponent of using natural, safe and inexpensive supplements whenever possible. I liked that prescriptive anti-fungals and my diet gave us quick results, but I always worried that we might be injuring someone's liver with these drugs. Fortunately, we did not, but in 1989 I didn't know that, nor did I know as much about using supplements that had anti-fungal properties.

In the early 1990s, I began speaking to lay audiences in cities that carried my radio program, and by the late 1990s I was speaking to crowded auditoriums filled with people who watched my show. All had health problems or knew a loved one with health problems, and they hoped that I could provide answers to their many questions. Not necessarily me, but my topic of interest, fungal diseases, had become a hot topic a decade later, and I was invited to begin teaching physicians what had been stored in my brain for 40 years. This was quite an honor and one that I continue to this day. In 2016, I was the keynote speaker at a mycotoxin symposium. A physician became fascinated with my work and challenged my hypothesis that fungus could cause so much illness. He began testing nearly all of his patients for the presence of fungus and found that over 75% had active, disease-causing fungus growing in their bodies. His practice is much different than it was before our meeting. He recently told me that The Kaufmann Diet alone represents 70-80% of his recommendations. He is using natural supplements like Neem, Horopito plant and caprylic acid (to name very few) in addition to the Kaufmann Diet with great success. He and I have become friends and share conversations often. I continue to refer people to him who I feel would ordinarily go to physicians that were unaware of the ability of fungal mycotoxins to injure and kill human beings. Without knowing the cause of an illness, we are relegated to spending the rest of our lives running to doctors' offices and pharmacies. Sound familiar?

There are thousands of anti-fungals available, including vitamin C, amino acids, fish oils and foods, including fruits and vegetables. *Simply concentrate on eating what fungus does not, and you should be fine.* If you are gradually improving (more range of motion, reduced pain and more energy), get excited; unfortunately, some scientists continue to point out that vegetables and dietary supplements do not cure anything, and perhaps they are correct. But a few weeks into this program, you are feeling so much better! Had you never tried it, you might be disappointed in yourself, but you did try it and are thus far satisfied. More of the same should really pay off for you as you continue to heal. You are to be congratulated!

In the end, a few weeks down the line you are either going to clearly indicate fungus as the cause of your fibromyalgia and/or fatigue or rule it out. Now that you know options exist, failure to try defines failure most accurately. Take a moment and read this medical work up by Lynn Jennings, MD. She is yet another physician that I introduced to fungal diseases long ago. I consider her a dear friend. This is a real case study done several years ago.

Fibromyalgia and Fatigue Case Study

By Lynn Jennings, M.D.

Thank Goodness for Summer Vacation

I have probably said this before; I am one of those people that actually loved going to school. Are you surprised? I love learning new things. Teachers will always have a special place in my heart. Who today would disagree when I say that schools are sometimes the most dangerous places to work? It is not for the reason you think. Read on...

For legal purposes I must give a disclaimer: This case study is for educational purposes only. I am using it to show you how a typical patient presents and the things I consider when I make a diagnosis. The patient's name has been changed to protect her identity. I practice integrative/alternative medicine, and my recommendations for treatment are often considered outside traditional practice. It is not my intent to criticize or denounce traditional medicine. I am merely providing an alternative opinion. Most importantly, the information provided here should not be used as a substitute for an examination and/ or treatment by a licensed health care provider.

Presenting illness:

Mrs. July is a 45 year old white female who presented to the clinic for an alternative medical consultation. She stated that she has "all over" body pain. The last time she felt good was 25 years ago. Simply put, Mrs. July has multiple medical problems which she believes are related to chronic fungal infection, and she has been unable to find a local doctor to treat her.

Past medical history:

Mrs. July has a history of migraines. She was diagnosed in 1999 with fibromyalgia. She has a history of gastro-esophageal reflux/irritable bowel syndrome. Mrs. July has degenerative disc disease of lumbosacral spine. She has problems with recurrent chest pain and an irregular heart beat.

Medications:

Mrs. July is on the following medications for pain and muscle spasm: Baclofen, Lidoderm patch as needed, Percocet and Darvocet. She is on the following medications for gastrointestinal problems: clonazepam, dicyclomine as needed, Phenergan as needed, Zofran as needed and ranitidine as needed. She is using a topical antibiotic gel (clindamycin) for acne control. She is using Lunesta as needed for insomnia and Lasix as needed for edema. Mrs. July has recently taken a short course of Diflucan (prescription anti-fungal) for a vaginal yeast infection.

Supplements/Vitamins:

Mrs. July is taking a number of vitamins and supplements including the following: caprylic acid, zinc, garlic, Estroven, Colace, biotin, cranberry, psyllium, melatonin, Immune Formula, Miralax as needed, vitamin C, vitamin B12, calcium, coenzyme Q10, vitamin D, B complex vitamin and a multivitamin.

Allergies:

Mrs. July has multiple medication allergies including metoprolol, flecainide, nortriptyline, verapamil, Imitrex, CartiaXT, Ambien, Effexor, Reglan and cephalosporin. She is allergic to MSG (monosodium glutamate) and peanuts.

Past surgical history:

Mrs. July had a tonsillectomy (1968), cholecystectomy (gallbladder removal) and hysterectomy with removal of one ovary (1999). She has had multiple lipomas (fatty tumors) excised from her back in 1987 and 1988. She has undergone wisdom tooth extraction with resultant nerve problems. Mrs. July has had ablation surgery on her heart for premature ventricular contractions (arrhythmia) in 2009. She underwent a bladder distention and bladder biopsy (1991). In February 2010 she underwent extensive lumbar spinal surgery.

Social history:

Mrs. July is married. She works as an elementary school teacher. She does not smoke and rarely drinks alcohol. Of note, Mrs. July works in a school that has been determined to have mold problems. The building where she works has had mold remediation with the exception of her classroom and one other. She has been told that her classroom is okay. Her daughter also had problems with mold from the same building.

Review of systems:

After her third pregnancy, Mrs. July developed uterine prolapse and was treated with antibiotics (amoxicillin) for three months. In 2008, Mrs. July was diagnosed with a viral gastrointestinal illness. A short time afterwards she developed a migraine and she gave herself an Imitrex injection to try and stop it. Unfortunately, Mrs. July had a reaction to the Imitrex injection with sharp chest pain and aching in her arms and neck. She was seen by a physician and was told that the viral illness had damaged her heart, causing an irregular heart beat known as premature ventricular contractions (PVCs). These premature ventricular contractions were causing such a problem that Mrs. July underwent a cardiac procedure known as ablation of the accessory pathways. Ablation involves passing an electric current to the very small area of the heart where the irregular beat originates and cauterizing (burning it). This procedure is done to stop the source of the irregular beats. Despite this procedure, Mrs. July continues to have episodes of sharp pain in her chest with radiation to her back as well as aching in her neck and arms.

In January 2010, Mrs. July developed a strep infection of the throat. In February 2010, she underwent spinal surgery on her lumbar spine. As a complication of the surgery she developed a methicillin resistant staph infection which was treated with tetracycline. Mrs. July states that she developed "all over" body pain after three days on the tetracycline.

She was able to talk her doctor into giving her four days of Diflucan and one week of Nystatin. Mrs. July reports that during the first few days of anti-fungal treatment she was very sick, but this improved. She followed the Kaufmann Diet and was feeling better. She stopped following the Kaufmann Diet because of travel and eating out. Since then, her pain has worsened.

Mrs. July reports that she is having problems with her hair falling out, fibrocystic breast disease, toenail fungus and feeling off balance. She has had kidney stones in the past. With regards to her recent back surgery, Mrs. July is wearing a spinal bone stimulator four hours a day and she will need to do this for nine months.

Mrs. July has been told that she has bursitis in both of her hips. She states that her orthopedic surgeon wants to inject steroids into both of her hips. She has received epidural steroid injections into her back and most recently (April 2010) she received a steroid injection in her hip. In June, she developed a yeast infection and was treated with 4 days of Diflucan. It has been suggested to her that she has an auto-immune disorder.

Physical exam:

Blood pressure: 130/89, Pulse: 104, Height: 5'9", Weight: 214 lbs.

Significant findings on physical exam include bilateral suborbital edema and scalloping of her tongue. She has some edema of her right and left lower legs. Her skin is dry and some of her toenails are thickened and yellow. She is noted to have trace beta carotenemia of the soles of her feet and spasm of the muscles in her back. The remainder of her exam was unremarkable.

Laboratory:

Vitamin D, 25-hydroxy: 25.6 ng/ml (normal values 32-100 ng/ml)

Discussion:

What would be your diagnoses? If I were practicing traditional medicine I would say that Mrs. July has multiple chronic medical diseases. By traditional standards I would be correct. But knowing what I do know, it is hard to pretend that that is the whole story. What I believe to be true is actually less complicated than saying Mrs. July has multiple, discrete and unrelated, chronic medical illnesses.

What if I say Mrs. July has chronic fungal infection? The underlying, chronic fungal infection has manifested as the signs of chronic medical disease such as chronic pain, arrhythmia, kidney stones, fibrocystic breast disease, fibromyalgia, irritable bowel syndrome, migraines, toenail fungus, low thyroid metabolism, bladder problems, vaginal yeast infections and arthritis. Did I miss something? I did not include her herniated discs/degenerative disc disease, but I did include her arthritis.

Unfortunately, some of her problems are as a result of traditional medical treatment. For example, Mrs. July has a hormonal imbalance as a result of her hysterectomy.

We can all agree that Mrs. July has a chronic fungal infection. Based on her history, this is a long-standing problem. She has not felt well for at least 25 years by her own reporting. So how did she get to this point? There are several ways that fungi can gain access into our bodies.

The first is by inhalation of fungi or its spores through our respiratory tract. Mrs. July works in a school building that has been identified as having mold. She reported that the school has undergone mold remediation except in her classroom and another. I am only guessing, but I suspect that it took quite awhile to recognize the mold problem. This implies that she has been breathing in spores and fungi over a long period of time (as are the children). The fact that mold was recognized as a problem probably means that there was quite a bit of mold visible to the naked eye. I do not know how old the building in question is, but the term *sick building* could apply here. Advances in architectural technology have allowed builders to create tightly sealed structures to keep out dust and pollen. Because of the tight seal, moisture can unfortunately collect and set up the perfect environment for fungal colonies to grow. In the case of accidental flooding from broken pipes or other causes, this tight seal can make it difficult for the building to dry out completely.

Second, fungi can gain access to our bodies through open places or cuts on our skin or through our skin. Most people have had a case of athlete's foot or toenail fungus. It is easily spread by contact. Mrs. July reports problems with toenail fungus.

The third and major route of infection with fungi is through our gastrointestinal tract. We can eat foods that are contaminated with fungus, or we can take antibiotics which promote the growth of fungus. Before you say I do not eat foods that are spoiled, and I throw away cheese or bread if it is moldy, let me ask you a few questions. Do you eat corn? Do you eat peanuts? Do you eat breads? Do you drink alcohol? All of the above are either contaminated with or are made with fungi. Corn is one of the worst offenders. It is known to be frequently contaminated with fungus. The government inspects corn for the presence of aflatoxin, which is a deadly mycotoxin produced by fungi that infest corn. The government checks for the amount of aflatoxin present, and if it is too high, then the contaminated corn is not allowed to be used for human consumption. I wish it stopped there, but it does not. Depending on the level of aflatoxin present, it may be used to feed cattle. Or, if it is too high for consumption by cattle, it can only be used to manufacture alcohol.

Mrs. July has had to take multiple courses of antibiotics throughout her life. With her history of bladder problems, as a doctor I know that she would have received multiple courses of antibiotics for a bladder infection. She has had a tonsillectomy which is usually preceded by multiple courses of antibiotics to treat the tonsillitis. Most recently, she received antibiotics for treatment of her methicillin resistant staph infection. Mrs. July states that her all over body pain began shortly after taking tetracycline.

Mrs. July's multiple drug allergies and irritable bowel syndromes are all consistent with fungal overgrowth of the gastrointestinal tract (leaky gut). In our gastrointestinal tract (as well as the rest of our bodies), there is a normal balance of human cells, bacteria and fungi. Normally the lining of the small and large intestines provides a semi-permeable barrier which prevents toxins, large molecules of food, bacteria and yeast from passing through to the tissues of the body and into the bloodstream.

There are a number of ways that this normal balance can become disrupted. One of the most common ways you can disrupt this balance is to eat foods that are contaminated with fungus such as corn, peanuts and grains. Another common way is through the use of antibiotics. When you are given an antibiotic, the antibiotic will kill off bad bacteria; this is what it is supposed to do. Unfortunately, you get more than you bargain for; antibiotics are nonspecific, and they will kill off good bacteria as well as bad bacteria.

Fungi are opportunistic; when the good bacteria of the GI tract are killed, this leaves a vacancy. Fungi that are present will grow to fill the vacancy left by the bacteria. We call this by several names: fungal overgrowth, leaky gut, dysbiosis or intestinal hyper-permeability. I am not saying that you should not take antibiotics, but this is one of the scenarios in which the gastrointestinal tract can develop this problem. When fungal overgrowth is present, the normal barrier lining the GI tract is disrupted at a microscopic level. The spaces between the cells lining the intestines get too large. Toxins, protein molecules, bacteria and fungi (yeast) are able to enter into the body and bloodstream that ordinarily should not.

Most people do not realize that 80% of your body's immune system is located in the tissues surrounding your gastrointestinal tract. This is known as the gastric-associated-lymphatic tissue (GALT).

When these protein molecules, bacteria and fungi enter the tissues surrounding the intestinal tract, the immune system (GALT) sees these as foreign invaders and begins to attack. This attack is called an inflammatory response. With chronic fungal overgrowth, you have chronic inflammation. Chronic inflammation is considered to be the underlying cause of many common, chronic medical conditions such as coronary artery disease, atherosclerosis, arthritis and auto-immune disorders.

The problem with leaky gut does not stop there. When it is present, our body also loses some of its ability to absorb nutrients properly from foods. This can lead to malnutrition as well as vitamin deficiencies. When talking about vitamin deficiency, I do not mean a severe deficiency as can occur when a patient has severe vitamin C deficiency like scurvy. What I am talking about is a relative vitamin deficiency; you have enough to prevent a vitamin deficiency disease but not enough to be at optimal health.

With regards to treatment, I have recommended that Mrs. July begin on a course of prescription anti-fungals, ketoconazole and Nystatin. I have recommended that she start on replacement probiotics, which are the replacement bacteria for her GI tract, and glutamine which will nourish the probiotics. The goal is to re-establish the normal lining of the gastrointestinal tract. Diet is absolutely essential for Mrs. July. She felt better when she was on The Kaufmann 1 Diet in the past, and I am recommending that she start back on it again

As a result of her dysbiosis, Mrs. July is suffering from relative vitamin deficiencies. Even by traditional medical standards, she has a vitamin D deficiency. I have recommended that she start on Vitamin D3 replacement, and I have recommended a course of specific vitamins and supplements to support her heart, muscles and metabolism. Based on her physical exam and symptoms I also believe that Mrs. July is suffering from hypothyroidism. I have started her on a thyroid replacement as well as iodine replacement.

Hopefully, with the above regimen and a summer vacation break from the school building, Mrs. July will be able to regain some of her health. We will see if her health continues to improve with the start of the next school year.

It would take a book or two to really explain how fungi and their mycotoxin could cause all of Mrs. July's medical problems. Fortunately, there are some books which do just that. For those of you who are interested in learning more about the connection between fungal infection and chronic medical disease, I recommend *The Fungus Link* Vol.1-3 by Doug Kaufmann.

Blessings,
Lynn Jennings,MD

Thank You, Dr. Jennings!

How and When to Start Thinking Fungus
for Your Fibromyalgia/CFS

The Chinese philosopher, Laozi, once stated that the journey of a thousand miles begins with the first step. How many times I have applied that logical first step in my life. You may wish to schedule this, because the first week may be a difficult one for you. During this period, you may notice more flare-ups, pain and fatigue. Why? You likely have awoken a sleeping giant inside your body; the giant was totally satisfied parasitizing your body for its own survival. You've fed it well for many years, and now that it is being starved, it is going to let you know of its displeasure in no uncertain terms!

Some of you may be so thrilled that there may be hope, you will just dig in and start today. Long term, you will find that an amazing thing happens. Depending upon the tissues affected and how deeply this parasite has grown inside of you, you may experience what many do: three days of knowing you have beaten it, followed by a day or two of exacerbation of the exact symptoms you are trying to fix even though you've been careful with the diet. Do not give up. It seems that fungi die off in chunks rather than in one fell swoop. You have suffered for a long time, so do not trust that the germs responsible for your suffering are going to vacate in a week or two. The wonderful thing about this entire program is that in a very short experimental period, you will know if you are on the right track of isolating the cause of your misery. Yes, it may take months to finally see the light at the end of the proverbial tunnel, but before reading this chapter, had you ever thought a light existed?

CHAPTER 10

I Don't Have a Fungal Problem! I Have Cancer!

The three-word phrase that frightens most people when it comes to doctor visits is, "You have cancer." If you have heard those words or have a loved one who has, this chapter like the others that precede it are meant to teach and comfort you. Simply put, poisonous fungal mycotoxins are well documented as a cause of cancer, yet these facts continue to elude our brightest and best scientists. I will explain this to you in detail in this chapter.

Again, let me remind you that I respect the book knowledge and treatment abilities that American doctors have, but unless mycology (the study of fungus) is taught in medical schools, which is currently not the case, our doctors are extremely limited in their scope of diagnosing or caring for cancer patients. As you will read, several fungal mycotoxins are listed by an accredited body known as the IRAC, or International Agency for Research on Cancer, as *possible*, *probable*, or *definite* cancer causing agents. Any physician who lacks this information lacks the entire picture of the cause of cancer.

Having said this, nothing compares to American doctors' abilities when it comes to transplantation surgery or emergency medicine procedures. If you need a kidney transplant, you're living in the right country. God forbid, if I'm in an auto accident today and break my arm, I am not going to put an organic, raw, non-GMO, gluten-free whole wheat poultice on my arm in lieu of seeking proper medical care. But how should you and I define "proper medical care" when it comes to our growing list of autoimmune diseases of which cancer is one of 135 such diseases? The standard of care for cancer patients is three-fold: surgery, chemotherapy and radiation. As I see it, that is a problem. You see, two of those three, chemotherapy and radiation, are themselves known cancer-causing agents. Not only do cancer patients have low immunity, but they also have cancer! Why is it that we have become complacent in further lowering their immunity with certain chemotherapy drugs and radium, both of which according to the IARC can cause low immunity and cancer?

The Most Common Female Cancers

According to the American Cancer Society (ACS) men get cancer more often than women, but women are more apt to survive it. The ACS has highlighted the 7 most common types of cancer that women can experience.

1. **Breast cancer** is the most common cancer that women will face in their lifetimes. The ACS recommends annual mammograms at age 45 for all women to detect breast cancer in its earliest stages.

2. **Colon cancers** are cancers of the colon and rectum and affect women with a history of inflammatory bowel diseases more often. Being overweight, eating a high fat diet, smoking and leading a sedentary lifestyle puts women at higher odds of getting colon cancer. Colonoscopy and stool testing is recommended.

3. **Endometrial cancers**, those affecting the lining of the uterus, are most common in women over the age of 55. Taking estrogen without progesterone and/or taking the medication Tamoxifen for breast cancer treatment or to lower your risk of breast cancer can increase the risk of endometrial cancer. Being overweight or having a history of polycystic ovary syndrome (PCOS) or having a history of hereditary non-polyposis colon cancer (HNPCC) can increase the risk of endometrial cancer.

4. Smoking cigarettes causes many cases of **lung cancer**, so simply stopping reduces your risk of lung cancer. Even non-smokers can get lung cancer however. The ACS recommends screening for certain people at higher risk of lung cancers.

5. **Cervical cancer** can affect women who are or have been sexually active. Since it is passed during sex, cervical cancer occurs in women who have had the human papilloma virus, or HPV. The risk for this cancer increases in women who smoke, have HIV or AIDS, have poor nutrition and those who do not get regular Pap tests. Pap testing is recommended every 3 years for women beginning at age 21.

6. **Skin cancer** occurs more often in fair skinned women, especially those with blond or red hair. Melanoma is a type of skin cancer that occurs more often in those who had bad sunburns as children or have a family history of melanoma. Broad-spectrum sunscreen protection of SPF 30 or higher, sunglasses, hats with brims and long sleeve shirts are recommended as preventive measures. Tanning beds and/or tanning lamps should be avoided. Having routine skin examinations done is recommended.

7. **Ovarian cancer** occurs more often as women age. At risk women include those who have never had children, who are infertile or had their first child after the age of 30. A history of hereditary non-polyposis colon cancer (HNPCC), ovarian cancer or breast cancer also increases the risk of ovarian cancer. It is advised that woman who have belly swelling, gas, loss of appetite, bloating, experience abdominal or pelvic pain and who feel the need to urinate often, if experienced for a few weeks, visit their doctor as these may be early signs of ovarian cancer.

Mind you, this information on cancer comes directly from the American Cancer Society and not me. This book has already expounded on my sentiments of the role of fungus in these and other cancers. Let me take a few moments and teach you a bit about fungal mycotoxins' role in breast cancer, since it seems to be the one cancer that occurs most often in women. With all due respect to fund raising organizations, jogging for a cure, while certainly generating hundreds of millions of research dollars, has yet to identify why it exists or how to fix it. That is because our brightest and best researchers are looking to pharmaceutical companies to end this terrible disease. Since they haven't, we need to look in a different direction.

One of the more exciting discoveries for breast cancer patients was made in the 1980s, and it is relevant to this book. It involved a researcher named Ross C. Donehower, M.D. and his colleagues at the John Hopkins Oncology Center, who described their discovery of *paclitaxel* as, "...a unique plant-derived substance that stops tumor growth."

As it turned out, it was the Pacific Yew Tree that harbored Paclitaxol and several new synthetic drugs, two of which were Taxol and Tamoxifen. These were developed thanks to the Johns Hopkins researchers. To this day, these drugs are used with good success by cancer patients. What you don't know (and I doubt the good Johns Hopkins researchers ever knew), is that Taxol and Tamoxifen both kill fungus! Plants have anti-fungal phenolic compounds, and the Pacific Yew tree is no exception. I recall the hype after their discovery decades ago as the drug industry scrambled to synthesize the Pacific Yew tree extracts that made these natural plant anti-cancer compounds a patentable drug. By 1992, at least 30 academic research teams were working on making a chemical that worked as well as the tree extract itself. Since natural substances cannot be patented, you see why chemicals are being added to them as a means of protecting their discoveries.

Breast Cancer Thoughts: An Ounce of Prevention...

For just a moment, turn back to chapter 2 and read the opening pages. In them, I state that fungal mycotoxins are known to disrupt our hormone-producing (endocrine) system, most notably altering estrogen. That is a huge and completely relevant statement when it comes to cancer of any type but particularly breast cancer. I read with great interest an article that appeared in the August 15, 2017 issue of U.S. News and World Report written by Elaine K. Howley. The title, "*Can Endocrine Disrupters Elevate Risk of Breast*

Cancer?" left me hoping that someone would finally implicate a little-know estrogenic mycotoxin called zearalenone in breast cancer. It did not, because few people know that the fungus that makes this poisonous mycotoxin, *Fusarium*, even exists. For Elaine to miss it in her article is certainly understandable. She did use the words, "*synthetic (manmade) estrogens*, in her article, but referred only to DDT (a pesticide that has been banned for decades) and bisphenol A (BPA), which is a compound found in many plastics. But for our entire medical community to miss that the "elephant in the examination room" is a human estrogen-mimicking mycotoxin called zearalenone is truly incomprehensible.

Many studies show that as post-menopausal levels of estrogen increase, so does the risk of breast cancer. But doesn't menopause occur as a result of stopping the production of estrogen? If so, why would a 55 or 60-year-old female be at risk of both elevated estrogen levels and breast cancer? Might it have to do with exposure to this human estrogen-mimicker called zearalenone? Are we humans even exposed to it? To answer these questions, I'm going to refer to a website called Breast Cancer Prevention Partners, or bcpp.org. It used to be called the Breast Cancer Fund, and I am a fan of theirs. Here are some direct quotes from their website on the link between breast cancer and the fungal mycotoxin, zearalenone. The scientific references have been left out of the text, but they are listed on their website [1].

- *An important metabolite (breakdown product) of zearalenone is zeranol, a compound that is also produced as a synthetic compound (brand name Ralgro) and is largely used in the U.S. beef industry to increase growing speeds of the animals used for meat. Zearalenone and zeranol mimic the natural estrogen estradiol. Both compounds can stimulate growth and proliferation of human breast tumor cells in vitro at potencies similar to the effects of estradiol.*

- *Zeranol is a synthetic version of zearalenone, a natural chemical that is produced by the fungus, **Fusarium**. In vitro, zeranol stimulates growth and replication of human breast tumor cells that are sensitive to estrogen at rates similar to those induced by the*

natural hormone estradiol and the known carcinogen diethylstil-
bestrol (DES).

- Zearalenone can be found in many agricultural products, including cereals, mixed feeds, and rice. It may also be found in meat,
eggs, dairy and other products from animals that have consumed
the contaminated feed. Corn is the most commonly contaminated
crop, and high levels of zearalenone have been found in girls who
consume higher levels of popcorn. Zeranol is found in the meat of
U.S. and Canadian beef cattle treated with the drug. Studies have
shown the potentially damaging effects on abnormal cell growth
to be significant even at levels of zeranol that are almost 30 times
lower than the then-current FDA-established limit in beef of 150
parts per billion

- Studies have shown that zeranol is comparable to the natural
estrogen estradiol in its ability to transform normal human breast
cells into cells showing signs of early cancer development. Some
studies showed that adding zeranol to cultured breast epithelial cells resulted in a five-fold increase in volume compared to
non-zeranol-treated control cells. Preliminary data indicate that se-
rum (blood plasma) from zeranol-treated beef cattle can stimulate
the proliferation of normal breast epithelial cells and the transfor-
mation of breast tumor cells in vitro.

- Young girls are especially vulnerable to the health effects of
zeranol due to concerns about links between early puberty and
later-life breast cancer.

In an effort to remain unbiased, please know that our FDA approved
the use of Ralgro (zeranol) long ago and contends that its inclusion
in our meat supply is harmless. Although the website drugs.com lists
these precautions for Ralgro usage to farmers who use it:

Precautions
Not for use in breeding herd replacements or lactating dairy animals.
Edema of the vulva and udder, teat elongation, rectal and vaginal
prolapse, and signs of estrus may occur when heifers are implanted.

Delayed testicular development may occur in young males. To avoid difficulty in castration, young males should be castrated at the time of implanting.

The FDA (fda.gov) labels Zeranol, or Ralgro, as safe. Here is an except regarding the use of steroid hormone drugs in our meat supply:

These steroid hormone drugs are typically formulated as pellets or "implants" that are placed under the skin on the back side of the animal's ear. The implants dissolve slowly under the skin and do not require removal. The ears of the treated animals are discarded at slaughter and are not used for human food. Using scientific data, FDA establishes the acceptable safe limits for hormones in meat. A safe level for human consumption is a level of drug in the meat that would be expected to have no harmful effect in humans based on extensive scientific study and review.

All approved steroid implant products have a zero day withdrawal. This means that the meat from the animal is safe for humans to eat at any time after the animal is treated.

How do you know if hormones like estrogen and progesterone are fueling breast cancer? Doctors will have your biopsy sent to specialists who will determine if it is hormone receptor positive (HR+). If it comes ER+, which an alarming 80% of breast cancer biopsies do, it is estrogen positive. Given the propensity for zearalenone to mimic human estrogen, I've got to wonder why no one has questioned this mycotoxin-derived meat additive as a cause of HR+ breast cancer, especially when the synthetic, pharmaceutical-made zearalenone, called zeranol, or Ralgro is many time more potent than the already poisonous mycotoxin itself.

Meat has been thought to cause many cancers for many years, but is it really the meat causing the cancer? Or, is it the meat additives (like antibiotics and growth hormones) that are cancerous? The purpose of this book is to educate you. Based on the issues covered, you must decide for yourself the route you choose to take now that you are armed with this information.

In chapter two, you also read that mycotoxins like zearalenone can suppress your immune system. With immunity down, we become vulnerable to opportunistic infections. Fungi are opportunistic germs and take advantage of our declining immunity whether it is mycotoxin-induced or part of the natural aging process.

I often think of how difficult it must be for cancer patients to trust their physicians as they observe their condition worsening. Some don't, but I'd imagine that most do. Please know that if you feel that you are worsening, this is not your doctor's fault as mycotoxicoses, or diseases caused by fungal mycotoxins, are not taught in medical school. Remember also that we must all be responsible for the decisions we make. Later in this chapter, you will see that the decision Alisa made may have saved her life, and it was her decision alone rather than her doctor's decision to make. She was fortunate to have such a supportive doctor.

I worked with many doctors' cancer patients who seemed to be failing with traditional cancer therapies. When I began to talk about diet, exercise (sweating) and nutritional supplements, most wanted me to know that their doctors disagreed with this approach. Often I heard, "My doctor says diet doesn't matter," or, "My doctor says that immune-building supplements should be avoided when you have an autoimmune disease like cancer." To you and me, logic might dictate that since their cancer was worsening, they needed to be more open-minded about change more than anything else. They were fearful, and I understand that, since they placed their hope in their doctor's hands who, in turn, placed his hopes in the pharmaceutical companies' hands. Sometimes, this approach does work effectively. Just to balance the scales, if the months or years with your cancer doctor have proven fruitful, and the cancer is improving, then stay on course! But the same thing might be said about alternative recommendations, if you feel that the traditional therapies are failing you. I am 100% comfortable with the decision that you and your loved ones make, but please share that decision with your doctors.

The next question facing cancer patients is that of cancer recurrence. Not knowing what caused this cancer might have you in a bind if the cancer comes back, whereas knowing that your moldy home or years of taking penicillin or previous alcohol problems—each exposing you to mycotoxins—would have you working on permanently eliminating the cause more than worrying about its recurrence. There is strength in knowledge!

Early in this book, I spoke about my being honored to speak, not only to lay audiences during the past 30+ years, but more recently to physician audiences. Watching faces during my lectures on fungus and its role in cancer has been educational for me. Lay audiences' faces tend to light up like Christmas trees when I mention that antibiotics increase the risk of many cancers. Physicians, however, often remain unresponsive. I would be too if I had just learned that my prescription pad might have played a role in this illness.

Honestly, those who absorb my talks and then implement changes with their patients are quite possibly changing their patients' lives, and some are eager to tell me about this. Whereas one told me that he is now using an intravenous anti-fungal drug on his cancer patients, another apprised me that he and a pathologist friend had discovered a fungal tissue in a breast cancer biopsy. Reports like these continue to fuel my fascination with the role of fungus and their poisonous mycotoxins in the disease we call "cancer."

References:
(1) https://www.bcpp.org/resource/zeranol-and-mycoestrogens/

The Role of Fungal Mycotoxins in Cancer: 2016 Cancer Symposium Presentation

Just the Facts, Ma'am!

At the end of 2016, I was honored to be asked to speak to physicians at a cancer symposium. The title of my talk was *The Role of Fungal Mycotoxins in Cancer*. Excerpts from this presentation may help you better understand just how commonly we are exposed to disease-causing fungi and their role in cancer. After reviewing, you might justifiably begin to wonder if your cancer, or that of a loved one, might involve fungus. These slides are actual depictions of my presentation.

Slide #3

Upon completion of this session, participants will improve their physician competence and performance by being able to better understand the role of fungal mycotoxins in cancer. Physicians will learn of FDA-approved anti-fungal drugs that have been studied regarding their role in cancer. Prescribing these anti-fungal drugs and altering a cancer patient's diet may offer therapeutic benefits.

Slide #4

Question: Does fungus cause cancer or does it mimic cancer?
Answer: Both

Pathogenic fungi make poisonous byproducts called mycotoxins. Some are genotoxic carcinogens. Most fungi produce microscopic spores inside special, elongated cells or sacs called ascomycetes. Mycetomas are fungal infections characterized by localized swelling, abscesses, and tumor-like granules. *A mycetoma can clinically masquerade as squamous cell carcinoma.* [1]

Slide #5

The American Cancer Society defines fungal mycotoxins as "genotoxic carcinogens." [2]

Slide #10

Fungal mycotoxins can be one or more of the following: Carcinogenic, Tremorgenic, Teratogenic, Genotoxic, Neurotoxic, Nephrotoxic, Hepatotoxic, Hemotoxic, Cardiotoxic, Lymphotoxic, Endocrine Disrupting, Dermatotoxic and/or Immunosuppressive (most mycotoxins are immunosuppressive).

Slide #11

Fungal infections, including paracoccidioidomycosis, histoplasmosis, cryptococcocis, coccidioidomycosis, aspergillosis, mucormycosis and blastomycosis, can mimic both the clinical and radiological findings of lung cancer. [3]

Slide #13

At least 33 mycotoxins are known mutagens; ill effects of exposure range from annoying to life threatening. These are capable of causing disease and death in humans. [4]

Slide #15

Cancer researchers inoculate study animals with the mycotoxin, aflatoxin. Aflatoxins are very toxic and carcinogenic mycotoxins, produced by *Aspergillus* and *Penicillium* fungi. Post inoculation, animals should be diagnosed with *aflatoxocosis* or *mycotoxicosis*. Soon, the symptoms in these animals parallel cancer identically. But is it really cancer? *They were not inoculated with cancer.* They were inoculated with a known carcinogenic mycotoxin which induced DNA mutations.

Slide #16

"Aflatoxins produce acute necrosis, cirrhosis and carcinoma of the liver in a number of animal species; no animal species is resistant to the acute toxic effects of aflatoxins; hence it is logical to assume that humans may be similarly affected." – FDA.gov

Slide #17

A case series was presented of 27 patients initially diagnosed, both clinically and radiologically, with primary or secondary lung cancer. These later proved to be fungal infections and all 27 patients responded well to anti-fungal therapy. [5]

Slide #18

In the book, *Clinical and Immunologic Aspects of Fungous Diseases (1957)*, there are multiple references to fungus mimicking cancer. [6]

- Pulmonary Coccidioidomycosis is "suggestive of metastatic malignancy." (P. 11)
- Localized cutaneous Blastomycosis is "frequently mistaken for squamous cell carcinoma." (P. 115)
- Disseminated Histoplasmosis is "found to coexist with leukemia, lymphosarcoma, sarcoidosis and Hodgkin's disease much more frequently than is statistically justifiable based on coincidence." (P. 153)
- Disseminated Cryptococcosis "closely simulates neoplasm." (P. 175)

Slide #28

Sac (ascomycetes) Fungi

Aspergillus, Penicillium and Fusarium are each "ascomycete" fungi. These are a recently discovered class of fungi; 75%+ of all fungi are ascomycete fungi. Spores reproduce in a tightly woven sac where meiosis, mitosis and nuclear fusion take place. These include morels and some edible mushrooms, bakers yeast, brewers yeast, and truffles to name a few.

Slide #29

Cancer or Fungus?

- Each can thrive in a sac formation
- Each can metabolize nutrients in the absence of oxygen
- Each generates lactic acid
- Each depends on their hosts for sustenance, proliferation and reproduction
- Each thrive in the presence of sugar and die in the absence of sugar
- Both emit Volatile Organic Compounds (VOC's) that dogs can detect
- Both respond to anti-fungal medicines

Slide #36
Exposure to Fungus

• Most often fungal spores are ingested or inhaled
• Diet
• Medication
• Inhalation

Are your cancer patients eating fungal impregnated food, drinking alcohol, living in a moldy home or have they been on many rounds of antibiotics? *Each exposes them to fungal mycotoxins.*

Slide #37
Dietary Mycotoxin Exposure
"Mycotoxins are toxic fungal metabolites which are structurally diverse, *common contaminants of the ingredients of animal feed and human food...*" [7]

Slide #38
American grain supply is commonly contaminated with (fungal) mycotoxins. [8] Corn is universally contaminated with fumonisin and to a less degree, other fungi and their toxins [9]

Slide #39
Fungal Exposure: Diet and Alcohol
Saccharomyces (brewer's) yeast is the fungus, and the mycotoxin it makes is called alcohol. Other mycotoxins besides alcohol can also be introduced into these beverages through the use of mold-contaminated grains and fruits. *Producers often use grains that are too contaminated with fungi and mycotoxins to be used for table food*, so the risk is higher that you are consuming more than just alcohol in your beverage. [10] The International Agency for Research on Cancer (IARC) lists Alcohol as a group 1 (known) human carcinogen.

Slide #40
Fungal Exposure: Medication
Are penicillin and other antibiotics carcinogenic in humans? Penicillium is the fungus and the mycotoxin it makes is called *penicillin*. "Certainly physicians would not believe such a risk exists for penicillin, an antibiotic given to billions of humans. However, it is by definition a mycotoxin, and mycotoxins do cause cancer." – Dr. A. V. Costantini [11]

Slide #42
Various epidemiological studies have reported that frequent use of antibiotics significantly increases risk of prostate cancer [12], lung cancer [13], breast cancer [14], colorectal cancer [15] and non-Hodgkin's lymphoma [16].

Slide #43
Fungal Exposure: Inhalation
"In addition to *Histoplasmosis*, lung infections with *Aspergillus sp.* and other molds can also resemble lung cancer on CT scans and other lung imaging techniques." [17]

Slide #45
Repurposing the Clinically Efficacious Anti-Fungal Agent Itraconazole as an Anti-Cancer Chemotherapeutic
It has been previously suggested that Itraconazole (Sporanox) not only inhibits the Hh pathway through a key regulator of this signaling cascade, but it also inhibits angiogenesis. This paper ruled out that Itraconazole worked by inhibiting this pathway. Might the reason that Itraconazole works for cancer be the exact reason that it works for toenail fungus? It simply kills fungus. [18]

Slide #46
Anti-fungal Drug Stops Cancer from Metastasizing by Inhibiting Angiogenesis
Researchers at Johns Hopkins have discovered *to their surprise* that a drug commonly used to treat toenail fungus, Itraconazole (Sporanox), could also block the growth of new blood vessels commonly seen in cancers. [19]

Slide #52

An inexpensive anti-fungal drug slows tumor growth and shows promise as a chemotherapy for cancer; in trials on mice, thiabenda-zole decreased blood vessel growth in fibrosarcoma tumors by more than 50% and it also slowed the growth of the tumors to a crawl. [20]

Slide #55

Mycotoxin Deactivators and Supplements That Inhibit *In Vivo* Mycotoxin Proliferation

- Psyllium (binds mycotoxins)
- Activated charcoal
- Bentonite clay
- NAC
- Alpha Lipoic Acid
- Glutathione
- Curcumin
- Trans-Resveratrol
- Chlorophyll (chemo-protective)
- Zinc
- Garlic

Slide #56

Why Isn't This Known?

"Fungi are the cause of many outbreaks of disease, but are mostly ignored.

Fungi can cause a number of life-threatening diseases... Many people, scientists among them, are largely unaware." —American Academy of Microbiology [21]

Congratulations! You now have "physician insider information" of the fungus link to cancer. After reviewing these slides, aren't you more hopeful to see if this program might assist you, or a loved one, in either proving or ruling out fungus as the cause of cancer?

The years and many wonderful doctors' patients that I worked with taught me that there is no one-size-fits-all therapeutic program for every cancer patient. If there were, chemo and radiation would cure all cancer patients. The same is true for more natural approaches to assist cancer patients. I discovered that fungi are smart little buggers and they've existed far longer than we have. They know how to identify and defeat their chosen enemy, and they are extremely good at it. Unfortunately, you may have become their chosen enemy—as long as you enable them. You now know that these fungi can live in sac formations that can resemble cancer tumors.

Those who have had or will have a biopsy, please consider splitting the biopsy sample and having one half of it tested for cancer per your doctor's recommendation and the other half tested for fungus. If you had a biopsy, even 25 years ago, it is still wrapped in paraffin at the testing facility that originally diagnosed you. It is never too late to have that biopsy tested for fungus as long as you can get the sample sent to a laboratory (there are several of them that do fungal DNA testing) that specializes in fungal tissue testing. Generally, it takes longer to test for fungus, but it could be the most important lab test you will ever have!

References:
(1) Momin, Saira B, et al. "Mycetoma Clinically Masquerading as Squamous Cell Carcinoma." *Journal of Clinical and Aesthetic Dermatology*, w, no. w, Feb. 2009, pp. 26–31.
(2) Murphy, Gerald P., et al. *American Cancer Society Textbook of Clinical Oncology*. American Cancer Society, 1995.
(3) Gazzoni, Fernando F., et al. "Fungal Diseases Mimicking Primary Lung Cancer: Radiologic-Pathologic Correlation." *Mycoses*, vol. 57, no. 4, 2013, pp. 197–208., doi:10.1111/myc.12150.
(5) Guimarães, Marcos Duarte, et al. "Fungal Infection Mimicking Pulmonary Malignancy: Clinical and Radiological Characteristics." *Lung*, vol. 191, no. 6, 2013, pp. 655–662., doi:10.1007/s00408-013-9506-0.
(6) Wilson, J. Walter. *Clinical and Immunologic Aspects of Fungous Diseases*. Thomas, 1957.

(7) Wang, Jia-Sheng, and John D Groopman. "DNA Damage by Mycotoxins." *Mutation Research/Fundamental and Molecular Mechanisms of Mutagenesis*, vol. 424, no. 1-2, 1999, pp. 167–181., doi:10.1016/s0027-5107(99)00017-2.

(8) Etzel, Ruth A. "Mycotoxins." *Jama*, vol. 287, no. 4, 2002, p. 425., doi:10.1001/jama.287.4.425.

(9) Council for Agricultural Science and Technology (CAST). *Mycotoxins: Risks in Plant, Animal and Human Systems*. Task Force Report No. 139. Ames, IA. Jan 2003

(10) Council for Agricultural Science and Technology. *Mycotoxins: Economic and Health Risks*. Task Force Report Number 116. CAST. Ames, IA. Nov 1989

(11) Costantini, A V, and M D Qvick. *Etiology and Prevention of Prostate Cancer Hope at Last*. Fungalbionics Series, 2002.

(12) Tamim, Hani M., et al. "Association between Antibiotic Use and Risk of Prostate Cancer." *International Journal of Cancer*, 2010, doi:10.1002/ijc.25139.

(13) Zhang, H., et al. "Antibiotic Use and the Risk of Lung Cancer." *Cancer Epidemiology Biomarkers & Prevention*, vol. 17, no. 6, Jan. 2008, pp. 1308–1315., doi:10.1158/1055-9965.epi-07-2817.

(14) Tamim, H M, et al. "Risk of Breast Cancer in Relation to Antibiotic Use." *Pharmacoepidemiology and Drug Safety*, vol. 17, no. 2, Feb. 2008, pp. 144–150., doi:DOI: 10.1002/pds.1512.

(15) Wang, Jiun-Ling, et al. "Infection, Antibiotic Therapy and Risk of Colorectal Cancer: A Nationwide Nested Case-Control Study in Patients with Type 2 Diabetes Mellitus." *International Journal of Cancer*, vol. 135, no. 4, 2014, pp. 956–967., doi:10.1002/ijc.28738.

(16) Kato, Ikuko, et al. "History of Antibiotic Use and Risk of Non-Hodgkins Lymphoma (NHL)." *International Journal of Cancer*, vol. 107, no. 1, 2003, pp. 99–105., doi:10.1002/ijc.11356.

(17) Salhab, Khaled F, et al. "Growing PET Positive Nodule in a Patient with Histoplasmosis: Case Report." *Journal of Cardiothoracic Surgery*, vol. 1, no. 1, Apr. 2006, doi:10.1186/1749-8090-1-23.

(18) Pace, Jennifer R., et al. "Repurposing the Clinically Efficacious Antifungal Agent Itraconazole as an Anticancer Chemotherapeutic." *Journal of Medicinal Chemistry*, vol. 59, no. 8, June 2016, pp. 3635–3649., doi:10.1021/acs.jmedchem.5b01718.

(19) "Antifungal Drug Stops Blood Vessel Growth - 04/26/2007." *Johns Hopkins Medicine Health Library*, www.hopkinsmedicine.org/news/media/releases/Antifungal_Drug_Stops_Blood_Vessel_Growth.

(20) "Common Antifungal Drug Decreases Tumor Growth and Shows Promise as Cancer Therapy." *ScienceDaily*, ScienceDaily, 21 Aug. 2012, www.sciencedaily.com/releases/2012/08/120821094358.htm.

(21) "The Fungal Kingdom: Diverse and Essential Roles in Earth's Ecosystem, 2008." *American Society for Microbiology*, www.asm.org/index.php/colloquium-reports/item/4517-the-fungal-kingdom-diverse-and-essential-roles-in-earths-ecosystem.

Physician Testimonials

During the week of May 22-29 2017, I received two emails from physician friends. Both have to do with treating fungal conditions that may look like cancer. I received permission from both doctors to excerpt and republish their emails. I have deleted their names, but I assure you these are absolutely real, unaltered words from two physicians.

Family Practice

Dear Doug,

I hope that you are well.

I just want you to know that we got another new patient yesterday who saw me on your TV show.

I am now routinely using anti-fungals in my cancer cases, especially itraconazole. I have a case of a "brain met" that disappeared! Gamma knife treatment was cancelled!!!

Thank you for all that you do.

Oncologist

Doug,

I suspect that fungus is a factor in many cancers, and as a result I have made fluconazole IVs a core component of my integrative cancer protocols. Since adding this therapy, I have noticed increased reductions in tumor markers on lab testing as well as visible reductions in the size of palpable tumors in my breast cancer patients. While these results are likely due to a combination of treatments I provide, I believe that addressing possible fungal involvement is a key aspect of my approach.

In early 2018, I received communication from a social media viewer who became hopeful that I could help her when she heard me mention that in some cases cancer is being misdiagnosed. I know this sounds impossible to believe, but even when the lab confirms that the tissue was cancerous, it may not be, which is the case here.

Alisa lives in California and asked me what I would do in her situation. Alisa had a mass on her neck that was seen by a specialist who took a biopsy; she had been diagnosed with "aggressive, stage 3 non-Hodgkin's lymphoma." I referred her to a physician friend not far from her home, knowing that he was aware of my work and knew that fungus played a role in some cancers. A few months later, I received this overview email from Alisa.

Oct 2017, I discovered a lump on my neck. Had no pain or other symptoms, but it didn't go away.

The MRI did not look good. I immediately followed the Phase (Kaufmann) One Diet MORE CLOSELY; I stopped eating sugar, carbs & began eating "cleaner."

I was diagnosed with aggressive, stage three non-Hodgkin lymphoma, chemo was recommended, I said no.

God prepared me several years prior when I began watching Know the Cause with Doug Kaufmann. It truly opened my eyes to good health. I also watched a docu-series, The Truth About Cancer, that supported what Doug had shared.

The Lord opened doors and led us to the right people, a safe, reputable source of CBD Oil, Colloidal/Ionic Silver Water and the Essiac Tea. Doug also recommended a doctor and he was great! He recommended great supplements & Vit-C IVs, which I've done.

I also do Infrared saunas to detox.

On Wednesday, Oct 10, 2018, the PET scan revealed I'm in COMPLETE REMISSION, NO cancer! The Oncologist said I am his first patient with this "response" & this time was more interested in all that I was doing.

TO GOD BE ALL THE GLORY!!!

A few days later, I received this email from the doctor I asked her to see;

> *Hi Doug!*
>
> *I just saw Alisa today…B cell lymphoma gone, tumor neck gone, recent PET scan normal…oncologist shocked; she has been following your diet (long before I saw her) and my supplement recommendations…Warmly,*

Nothing prepares me for these amazing testimonials. I could fill this book just with cancer testimonials that I have received over the years. All of this leads me to believe that we are grossly over-diagnosing cancer in America. Why did Alisa suspect that her cancer has a fungal basis? Alisa told me that her prayers were answered before she ever called me for the name of a referral. That is a great place for all of us to start!

Based on your fungal exposure history, if you suspect that your cancer may have a fungal basis (read Your Spore Score in the appendix), or learn later from laboratory data that your tumor had fungal tissue in it, I would request anti-fungal drugs for a few weeks. As you read above in my lecture notes, Sporanox (Itraconazole) seems to work quite well at not only inhibiting cancer from spreading but also in killing cancer cells. For this reason, I'd ask my doctor for 21 days of Sporanox and thereafter get his permission to discontinue Sporanox in favor of using potent anti-fungal supplements like Sacred Frankincense Oil, Cat's Claw, Essiac Tea, Pau D Arco, Vitamin C and Lactoferrin to name a very few. I've always believed in rotating these, perhaps every 2 weeks, as fungi can outsmart our most powerful drugs and nutritional supplements. Also inquire about using intravenous vitamins like those in The Myer's Cocktail or others.

Far infrared saunas may also be useful, but talk to your healthcare provider about using this detoxifying device before starting it since he knows your medical history.

If you have found a fungal link or component of your cancer, it is imperative to find a physician who will offer his expertise in this area to you. Traditional cancer treatment might be the correct choice for some people, but perhaps not for all people especially if after reading this chapter you suspect a fungal cause of it. Never in your life have you had to make so many decisions and make them as though your life depended upon them. Now is the time for you to shine! Make wise choices based on wise scientific data from both sides of medicine. Yes, traditional medicine has much to offer, but so does alternative medicine. I hope this chapter has assisted you!

CHAPTER 11

I Will Change My Diet Under Two Conditions: The New Diet Tastes Great and I Feel Better!

In the preceding chapters, case studies and solutions offered, I have been building the case that it makes sense to think of fungus as a valid link to most every disease for which the cause remains unknown. In this chapter, I'm going to teach you about the Kaufmann Diets.

The Kaufmann Diets and Lifestyle are tools I have designed over the years to assist you in discovering if fungus may lie at the core of your health problems. For this reason, it is imperative that you share this diet and your desires to begin the diet with your licensed healthcare provider. Only he/she knows about your specific health problems and has examined you and followed your course of treatments with you.

My diet has evolved because my awareness and the food industry itself has evolved. Decades ago, I had no idea that there were 2500 variations of apples, but there are. I thought there were only three: yellow, green and red. I chose green apples and left out yellow and red, because I had read that yellow and red apples contained more fruit sugar than green apples. I wanted to limit sugar, because it fed fungus. Many years later, I learned that an apple's sugar content has little to do with why so many people did well on my diet. Apples, as it turns out, have an anti-fungal component called malic acid as long as they are unripe or green. Green apples were serendipitously the right choice! Until a few years ago, I had no idea that buckwheat and millet were seeds! I thought they were grains and as such should be eliminated on my diets. Decades into this I'm still learning. The food industry is also changing as they combine yeast and bacteria to ferment foods and as our desires to eat these foods increases. As you will read, deciding which of these foods is "fungus friendly" and which is not is made simple in this chapter.

Diet can be a very useful tool in your recovery for two reasons, the first being obvious. Feeling better a few weeks from now is the "brass ring" you've hoped for. The second reason can be equally rewarding. Your next visit to your medical specialist will prove that the years of misery you've spent have come to an end. In a short amount of time, dietary changes have made all the difference in how you feel. Witnessing your improvement will have him/her and thousands of other physicians across this great country questioning their lab tests and robotic prescription habits. Every one of us wants to help fellow man, and you just accomplished this by keeping your appointment with your doctor. I can't tell you how many physicians have "changed their tune" about diets when sick patients returned to their offices as well patients simply because they changed their diet! In essence, you showed your doctor what a $200,000 medical education didn't! More importantly, you became the seed planted in his brain as to a dietary link to so many of his patients' health problems. You may never hear it from your own doctor, but hundreds or thousands of his current and future patients will have you to thank for their recovery!

There have been many references to fungi behaving as parasites once inside the human body. As long as they have warmth and a constant food supply, they can set up permanent residence and start their families. In 1944, a medical textbook entitled *The Manual of Clinical Mycology* gave some very early references to yeasts' insatiable appetite for sugar once they are inside of us. (Remember that yeasts are single-celled fungi). Sugar comes in many forms in our diet, including breads, soda, pasta and breakfast cereals. In this book, five Duke University physician authors stated, quite simply, that if you wished to successfully defeat yeast once it has invaded your body, you must lower your dietary intake of sugars or carbohydrates. They said this in 1944! How I wish todays' finest medical specialists knew this, as it would unquestionably change their course of treatment; perhaps therein lies the obstacle. Doctor are taught to very quickly examine, diagnose and prescribe. These actions have become the very core of a $5,000,000,000,000 (yes, five trillion) annual business.

What Qualifies Foods to Be Listed on the Kaufmann Diets?

Foods must meet certain criteria to be included in the Kaufmann 1 Diet. A food must have a very low risk of being contaminated with fungus or mycotoxins. A food must not potentially feed a disease-causing fungal infection. Foods might also exhibit some sort of anti-fungal quality, as fresh fruits and vegetables do. Finally, since addictive eating patterns might also harm your health, during the early stages of this program, we ask that you avoid the food or foods that you cannot seem to live without, even if they are on the Kaufmann 1 Diet. Truly, food addictions might arise out of actually being allergic to certain foods. While this restricts many foods, it encourages many others that not only protect against fungi and mycotoxins but also promote health, nourishment and vitality.

In my youth, I wanted to be a doctor. But the Vietnam War (OK...and my grades) interfered with that desire. My career, however, has been a blessing to me and as it turns out, a blessing to many others as well. I have worked with thousands of people directly and hundreds of thousands, perhaps millions, indirectly via radio and TV shows, lectures, etc. If I have learned anything in the past 45 years it is that when it comes to a nutritional protocol, we each have our own, personal "food thumbprint." If 10 cancer patients followed exactly the same nutritional protocol and had exactly the same biochemistry and physiology to break those foods and supplements down into nutritive and waste components exactly alike and 10 were cured of their cancers, we could stop inventing cancer treatments. We would finally know the exact protocol to cure cancer! Our avocados, carrots and parsley might be identical, but we are not. Because we are all unique, one protocol will never work for every person and every disease. Therefore, it is imperative that you work with a doctor, be they naturopathic or traditional, that will enable you to become involved in your own nutritional treatment based on that unique biological thumbprint that only you have.

Can I Be a Partner in My Own Recovery?

For that reason, I must have this discussion with you before you begin this program. I now believe that most of you, but perhaps not all of you, will benefit from following the Kaufmann 1 Diet for a period of time. The purpose of carefully staying on this diet is simple. It may help you get and feel better, but more importantly, it will finally teach you why you have been sick. I believe that this diet has liberated tens of thousands of people, because they finally achieved what they sought in so many doctors' offices for so many years: *the very reason they were sick*. Consider also that you may be one of the millions of Americans suffering from a dietary disorder, be it food allergy, which I believe is caused by bad guy yeasts poking holes in our intestines or fungus. This diet avoids many of the foods that are highly antigenic (capable of causing an immune response) on the allergy scale, but it also starves a living parasite—fungus—from your body given the right amount of time.

Some of you may initially feel worse for a few days while on the Kaufmann 1 Diet. If you were anything like me, *I catered to my own fungal infections without even knowing they was there*. I fed them, kept my body at 98.6 degrees and provide all they needed to live in comfort. I was their slave and had no idea! Then, in 1972, I began starving them to death. It is not pretty, in that fungi are tiny, living organisms, and sometimes they retaliate when they are being starved! We would too, but their demise is considered a good thing! Why "awaken" them? I did it at 21 years old and am glad I did. I believe that the aging process should not be viewed as a symptom or disease process, yet it so often is, because we enable fungi a lifestyle that was fitting for a king for decades, thereby delaying their ability to attack us until we are older and less able to defend ourselves. Address it now, or it will address you later!

After going through a few days of bizarre symptoms, the improvement may begin as you continue to stick with the diet. Most people told me that on the morning of the 3rd or 4th day, they woke up knowing that we were finally on the right track. Gradually, they feel better and better and then, for some, out of nowhere, bizarre symptoms begin once again even though they carefully stayed on the diet. I have long felt that these intermittent flare-ups or recurrences were due to these parasitic fungi letting you know that they were not gone yet. While some people began getting better the day they started the diet, others noticed improvement on day 4 of the diet. Still others took a few weeks until they felt that the diet was finally offering them relief. Why the difference? I think two things ultimately determine your relief date. First, how deep is the fungal infestation in your body? Deeper fungal conditions, as I believe the autoimmune disorders tend to be, take longer to starve. The second thing to consider is whether your new diet is made up of organic, fresh foods, or chemically-sprayed and fertilized genetically modified foods (GMO). Although still superior to grains and alcohol, these chemicals may slow down your rate of recovery. Most of you will know with certainty within 30 days if you were eating the wrong foods to recover, but some may take up to 60 days.

This, of course, raises the all-important question as to how long you are required to be on the Kaufmann 1 Diet. I know people who were once very, very ill, and you could not pry them off of the Kaufmann 1 Diet if you wanted to. They have followed it for years with great success. They know that the diet helped them to conquer a very serious health problem, and they are never going to veer from this diet. Is it safe to follow for long periods? Decades ago, I defined this diet as a temporary and experimental fungus starvation diet. I tried to add enough wholesome foods to sustain the person nutritionally while starving and killing underlying fungi that had been responsible for their misery. That said, the Kaufmann 1 Diet offers its followers an excellent, nutritionally-sound, very diversified diet while offering the exact opposite to the fungi that have been causing your misery. *They die, you thrive!*

I do not know your particular health problems or your health history, so it is imperative that you check with your own doctor. To the best of my knowledge, I have never had a doctor deny a patient of trying the diet, but please let him/her make that decision with you.

You may already know that a food or two that I have allowed on the diet does not sit well with you, and for that reason, with a felt marker, cross out those foods now. Yes, the diet may seem restrictive initially, but your illness has also been restrictive. If a change in diet would help you improve, life itself might be less restrictive. Remember, thousands are living their life on this diet and are thriving. After your doctor's approval, try it and see it you are not among them!

Welcome to the yeast/fungal—and therefore mycotoxin—starving diet!

The Kaufmann 1 Diet

1. **Sugar/Sweeteners**
   Allowed: Stevia and Xylitol

   Excluded: No sugar is allowed during Kaufmann 1, including honey, agave or other "natural" sweeteners. Aspartame, saccharine and most other artificial sweeteners are not allowed on the diet.

2. **Fruit**
   Allowed: Green apples, berries, avocados, fresh coconut, grapefruit, lemons, limes and tomatoes

   Excluded: Virtually all other fruits are excluded on Kaufmann 1 usually due to the high fructose content

3. **Meat**
   Allowed: Virtually all fresh, minimally processed meats. These include, beef, lamb, bison, turkey, chicken, pork, venison, etc. This also includes fish such as salmon, tuna and shellfish. Wild-caught fish and grass-fed or pasture-raised meats are always preferable. Avoid conventionally raised meat and farmed fish whenever possible as added hormones may affect fungal proliferation.

   Excluded: Beware of meats that have been cured using sugar, processed meats or deli meats which often contain sugar and/or ingredients such as wheat, corn, etc. Avoid breaded meats as well.

4. **Eggs**
   Allowed: All eggs.

   Excluded: Egg substitutes. They are not real eggs even if they contain eggs.

5. **Dairy**
   Keep in mind that dairy foods are often allergy foods, so if you are allergic to dairy, consider other non-dairy products. As a general rule, dairy products that are high in fat are low in milk sugar, called lactose. As you consider using dairy products while on the Kaufmann 1 Diet, consider also any addiction you may have to dairy products. Do you eat them daily? If you are not allergic to dairy foods and you are not over consuming them currently, you can enjoy them minimally while on the Kaufmann 1 Diet. Know that while on

the Kaufmann Diets, cattle that were grass-fed and grass-finished provide, in my opinion, the best meat and milk. Again, it cannot be overemphasized that lactose intolerance does exist, as does dairy allergy. Books have been written on how dairy allergy can cause some of the very symptoms you may be having. If you choose to eat dairy products, even the listed ones, watch for symptoms afterwards, and progress very carefully.

Allowed: Many people are allergic to dairy products. If so, avoid them totally. Of concern in dairy products is milk sugar, called lactose. Generally, the higher the fat, the lower the lactose level. Eat in moderation.

Butter is obviously a high fat product, but as such, contains only tiny amounts of lactose.

Ghee (clarified butter)

Yogurt—Goat yogurt, in moderation, is OK. Live cultured dairy probiotics contain relatively little lactose. Try to get higher fat yogurt with live bacterial cultures.

Heavy Cream—The fat skimmed of the top of milk creates heavy cream and it is about 37% fat. It contains almost no lactose.

Whipping Cream—Unsweetened; can be made by whipping heavy cream.

Sour Cream—Look for varieties made from real cream. There are now many suppliers of lactose free sour cream.

Cream Cheese—This is a low lactose cheese. There are now many suppliers of lactose-free cream cheese.

Excluded: Milk, other cheeses, margarine or other butter substitutes.

Dairy Substitutes:
The list of dairy free cheeses and milk substitutes grows monthly. There are many on the market now.

Allowed: Goat, coconut, almond and hemp dairy substitutes are acceptable.

Excluded: Rice or soy dairy substitute products

A Word on Kefir and Kombucha

Kefir grains and Kombucha scobys are fermented products like yogurt, but whereas yogurt utilizes bacterial fermentation, kefir and kombucha both use bacteria and yeast in their fermentation process. Saccharomyces, the yeast in these products, is the same yeast that is used to make bread, wine and beer. Ethanol and acetaldehyde are produced by saccharomyces during the fermentation process. These are only produced in small amounts in each kefir and kombucha drink, but as beverages that are heavily promoted for their health benefits, many people drink kefir and kombucha on a regular basis. As you read in chapter ten, acetaldehyde is a known carcinogen. For this reason, I excluded these products on the Kaufmann Diets.

6. **Vegetables**

Allowed: Virtually all fresh, unblemished vegetables are allowed. Greens are heavily encouraged. Juicing fresh, preferably organic vegetables and spices is acceptable.

Excluded: Potatoes and sweet potatoes, legumes (including beans, peas and green beans). Mushrooms and corn are not vegetables and are not allowed.

7. **Beverages**

Allowed: Filtered water, fresh-squeezed vegetable juices, many teas, including but not limited to white, green, African Roobios (red), purple and guayusa tea, unsweetened almond milk, coconut milk, and various other nut milks. Do not sweeten.

Excluded: Most others, including all alcoholic beverages, coffee, regular black tea, sodas and flavored beverages.

8. **Grains**

Allowed: Pseudo-grains such as quinoa, amaranth, buckwheat and millet. These are actually seeds. Also, black rice—also known as forbidden rice—is not forbidden on the Kaufmann 1 Diet.

Excluded: Virtually all other grains are excluded. These include corn, wheat, oats, barley, rye, spelt and any foods containing these ingredients including bread, pasta, cakes, crackers and other processed foods.

9. Yeast Products and Fungal Foods

Allowed: None. Be careful of foods that are fermented using yeast.

Excluded: Virtually all products containing yeast are excluded from the diet including alcohol, bread, etc. Any type of fungus, such as mushrooms and truffles, or foods that might contain fungus, such as certain aged cheeses or fungal byproducts, such as myco-protein or nutritional yeasts, are to be avoided as well.

10. Vinegars/Fermented Food Products

Allowed: Unpasteurized apple cider vinegar. Know that all vinegars are acidic. I have found that because it is rich in the anti-fungal agent malic acid, unpasteurized apple cider vinegar, in moderation, is OK.

Excluded: Virtually all others, including other vinegars, most salad dressings or sauces, pickled vegetables or fruit and soy sauce.

11. Oils

Allowed: Many oils are allowed including olive oil, macadamia nut oil, coconut oil, grape seed oil, flax seed oil, etc. Cold-pressed, extra virgin and minimally processed oils are best.

Excluded: Most vegetable oils, hydrogenated oils, corn oil, peanut oil, truffle oil and canola oil. Integrating rapeseed genes with the canola plant genes makes canola oil. Rapeseed oil contains a toxin called erucic acid. Even though canola oil contains low levels of erucic acid, I feel it is best to avoid this acid and genetically modified foods/oils until food chemists better understand what even tiny amounts of erucic acid really does to human cells and until they fully understand what modifying the genes of plants really does to human physiology.

12. Nuts & Seeds

Allowed: Most nuts and seeds are allowed on the diet, including walnuts, pecans, almonds, cashews, pumpkin seeds, etc. Know that cracked nutshells enable fungus to grow inside on the nut, so watch for broken shelled nuts. Be careful with sunflower seeds, because they can be contaminated with fungus. Nut butters are encouraged.

Excluded: Peanuts (including anything made with peanuts or peanut butter) and pistachios are to be avoided due to the likelihood of fungal contamination.

The Kaufmann 2 Diet

If your symptoms have improved while on The Kaufmann 1 Diet, some of you may want to add more foods into your diet and see if you continue to feel better. However, if you have a serious illness that has improved on this diet, you may wish to stay on The Kaufmann 1 Diet; improvement does not automatically translate to cure. This is yet another reason to share your successes on the diet with your healthcare provider. Further testing done by them may help educate them on the fungal basis of your illness.

The Kaufmann 2 Diet now introduces more foods into your diet. Be cautious when eating these new foods, and know that the Kaufmann 2 Diet may make you feel worse. If it does, reverting to The Kaufmann 1 Diet is easy and should have you feeling better quite quickly. For many, The Kaufmann 2 Diet means testing common foods that used to be in your diet often, like coffee and beans. Know that moderation is the key to success. If you find certain foods that bring back old symptoms, simply avoid those.

1. **Sugar/Sweeteners**
   You may experiment with minimal amounts of real Manuka honey that has an MGO (methylglyoxal factor) of 265+, in moderation as a trial. Manuka honey has antibacterial and anti-fungal properties, yet some cannot tolerate any honey, or they attempt to challenge it too early in their recovery.

2. **Fruit**
   Begin adding back fruits on occasion. Melons and bananas are discouraged. Babies do not require fruit juices, but fresh squeezed are OK. Bulk dried fruits are also discouraged, as they run a higher risk for fungal contamination.

3. **Meat**
   Same as Kaufmann 1

4. **Eggs**
   Same as Kaufmann 1

5. **Dairy**
   Lower lactose cheeses are fine to experiment with now. Cheeses that are very low in lactose are Cheddar, Parmesan (very high protein) and

Swiss cheeses. As a general rule, aged cheese is low lactose cheese. Older cheeses become hard because they lose their moisture content, and with that comes lower milk sugar. Hard cheese has much less lactose in it. Goat cheeses are generally fine.

6. **Vegetables**
   Allowed: You are now allowed to include sweet potatoes or yams and legumes including beans, peas, etc., in moderation. (Peanuts are still excluded.)

   Excluded: Regular potatoes. Mushrooms and corn are not vegetables and are not allowed.

7. **Beverages**
   Allowed: Since coffee is a bean, you may minimally experiment with coffee now, but be careful as fungal mycotoxins can be found in some coffee beans. Do not go overboard with coffee. Sweeten tea or coffee with stevia or xylitol.

   Excluded: Most others, alcohols, regular black tea, sodas and flavored beverages.

8. **Grains**
   Allowed: Oats and brown rice are allowed in moderation, because these tend to be less affected by fungus.

   Excluded: Virtually all other grains are excluded. These include corn, wheat, barley, rye, spelt and any foods containing these ingredients, including bread, pasta, cakes, crackers and other processed foods.

9. **Yeast Products and Fungal Foods**
   Same as Kaufmann 1

10. **Vinegars/Fermented Food Products**
    Same as Kaufmann 1

11. **Oils**
    Same as Kaufmann 1

12. **Nuts & Seeds**
    Same as Kaufmann 1

The Kaufmann Diet Compared to Other Diets

You Took Away All My Favorite Foods!

I realize this is a restrictive diet, at least at first. Recall that in the first chapter there was a section titled, *Eat Like Your Life Depends On It*. First, check with your doctor. If you are sick with fungal infection throughout your body, your life really may depend on lifestyle changes including diet. I have helped many people, including friends and family members, come back from the very brink of disease by following The Kaufmann 1 Diet. Eating the right foods and avoiding the wrong ones can help rid your body of fungi and their poisonous mycotoxins; this allows the natural, restorative process your body already possesses to work its magic and bring you back to vibrant life.

It is understandable, therefore, why so many people feel so much better while following The Kaufmann Diets. The point at which your symptoms begin getting better is the point at which this is no longer an experimental diet; the experiment worked. The Kaufmann Diets can safely become a lifestyle diet that can be followed and enjoyed for extended periods of time.

The Kaufmann Diet Compared to Other Diets

Because of the way diets have been marketed so heavily over the past four or five decades, most people equate diet with weight loss. If you need to lose weight, The Kaufmann Diet and Lifestyle may also help you do so; eliminating sugar and carbohydrates and getting good exercise will help you lose weight. However, if you need to lose a lot of weight and your doctor is suggesting a procedure or diet that might assist you more than The Kaufmann Diet, follow that advice. You might ask the doctor, however, if you can have 60 days to try this program before scheduling a weight loss surgery that might be recommended.

Think of The Kaufmann Diet as a filter for other diets. Take the foods that any other diet says you can have and compare them to the list of foods at the beginning of this chapter. You can discard foods on those diets that are not on the Kaufmann Diet list. For example, many popular diets include sweets and snacks that I do not agree should be commonly eaten when trying to get healthy or lose weight. Smaller quantities of bad choice foods are still bad choice foods, but you would not know it for all the labeling that proclaims this to be healthy or smart.

There are three specific diets that can get confused with The Kaufmann Diet. The first are the very low-carb diets including the famous Atkins Diet. I knew and really liked Dr. Atkins. His diet plan awoke a sleeping giant within the weight loss community decades ago, and I still consider him a pioneer. Cutting out many carbohydrates is not a bad way to start, but it fails to address things like peanuts, pistachios and the antibiotics or added hormones in chicken and beef that might have helped fungus grow in your body. I think Dr. Atkins had the right solution, but for the wrong problem.

The second is similar to the first. The gluten-free diet is currently en vogue as I am writing this book. Gluten is a protein that is packed into grain seeds along with carbohydrates. These are what the seeds eat to grow into stalks of grain. Recall that fungi also like to eat those carbohydrates. The grains that are avoided on the gluten-free diet are wheat, rye and barley. Since grains convert to sugars in our body and since grains are sometimes contaminated with fungal mycotoxins, the gluten-free diet might once again offer the right solution to the wrong problem. Many people are following the gluten-free diet and feel great, but what they do not realize is that it may not be the gluten in those grains that was causing their health problems, rather it may have been the fungal mycotoxins that contaminated those grains.

Have you ever tried the gluten free diet and thought it worked initially? Then, a few weeks later, WHAM! The old symptoms are back again despite being careful on the diet. Well, the problem for most gluten free followers is that both corn and sugar are gluten-free. Sugar feeds yeast and fungi, and corn seems to be very commonly contaminated with fungal mycotoxins. For many ex-followers, relief while on the gluten-free diet was short lived, and when the symptoms come back, people have no idea why. Now you know why!

The third is the popular paleo diet. The initial paleo diet and The Kaufmann 1 Diet are similar. In my opinion, one of the problems with the paleo diet is that it has been victimized by its own success. There appears to be several different versions of the paleo diet (ultimateplaeoguide.com), each approving of alcohol consumption. One version approves of eating white rice. Mushrooms are approved for eating without restriction on the paleo diet, but because they are fungus, they are eliminated totally on the Kaufmann Diets.

Paleodiet.com references the many variations of the paleo diet. While I disagree with drinking alcohol or eating rice or mushrooms, I can see how confusion abounds with so many variations and versions of the paleo diet in existence. Having said this, to a certain extent, the paleo diet is very much like the Kaufmann Diets, so it is plain to see why so many follow their own version of it and love it. Basically, if if you're eating to starve fungus, I'm all for it!

The Kaufmann Diets: Supplements

As our knowledge grows within the field of clinical nutrition, we as a society have learned that even the best diets for our bodies may be lacking in nutrients that provide optimum health or that are good for fighting fungus. At the same time, the world has gotten smaller, and we now know where to find plants that contain these very nutrients. The growth of the dietary supplement industry could not have come at a more fortuitous time for you.

35 years ago, the use of anti-fungals seemed to be limited to prescriptive drugs like Diflucan and Nystatin. But thousands of scientific studies have discovered that natural, plant-based supplements like cinnamon and resveratrol may have similar benefits. It sounds silly to say we now have these natural supplements, because they are mentioned in ancient texts like the Bible. It is more accurate to say that we now know that they tend to cleanse the body in much the same way that Diflucan and Nystatin do.

They are not alone. There are a wealth of supplements that either help stop fungus growth, restore damaged tissues or both. These are the supplements we recommend on the Kaufmann Diets.

Some Anti-Fungal Supplements

Pharmaceutical medicine has no shortage of chemicals designed to fight pathogenic fungal infections. These may be necessary in some circumstances, especially if you have an advanced disease. Remember that while your doctor may acknowledge that fungi do play a role in certain symptoms, he or she may likely disregard that some or all of your symptoms could be caused by fungus. Since pharmaceutical-grade anti-fungal medicines are available only with a prescription, the chances of your doctor writing you a prescription for one is low, unless he or she understands the fungus link to disease. Sadly, there is only a short list of practitioners who are well versed in this field of study. Be patient and continue your research in this area. Most, I have learned, bode well with natural supplements that have anti-fungal properties and may not require anti-fungal medications, but it is always best to ask your doctor and let him make that call.

There are a number of safe, natural supplements available—many of them foods themselves or food-derived—that may assist you in combating a fungal infection. There are volumes of literature written on the benefits of certain nutrients, and for a more comprehensive overview of anti-fungal supplements and nutrients, more research may be required. However, listed below are a few common, popular supplements that may assist in helping you fight a pathogenic fungal infection. It is recommended to rotate these supplements as part of your anti-fungal diet.

Two things are important to note: No one supplement ever seems to be effective alone. Anti-fungal supplements are most effective in the context of an anti-fungal program, including diet and exercise. Secondly, always consult your doctor before beginning a supplement or exercise regimen; some supplements can interfere with certain medications. Make certain that your body is ready to begin an exercise program by speaking to your doctor about this.

Cinnamon
Cinnamon has potent anti-fungal and anti-yeast properties. Some studies have shown that pharmaceutical grade (USP) cinnamon to be as or more effective than certain prescription medications at eliminating yeast. Cinnamon may also provide benefits for those trying to control blood sugar.

Oregano Oil
Oregano has been used for millennia as both food and medicine. Oregano oil is potently anti-fungal, but go slowly.

Olive Leaf
Studies done many years ago showed that the whole olive leaf is superior to certain extracts taken from the olive leaf like oleuropein. Sometimes, components of supplements are added in larger doses when the entire leaf is best. This is often done for marketing and sales purposes.

Grapefruit Seed Extract

GSE is a potent anti-microbial with a variety of uses. Its potency could be compared to that of a natural antibiotic. For this reason, it is a good idea to also take probiotics with GSE.

Tea Tree Oil

Tea tree oil is not for use internally, but this oil may be beneficial for people suffering with topical (skin) fungal infections.

Fish Oil

Fish oil has gained much mainstream attention for its cardiovascular and brain benefits, but the omega 3 fats inherent in fish oil also possess anti-fungal properties. This supplement does not need to be rotated but can become a part of your every day regimen.

Caprylic Acid

This powerful fatty acid derived from coconut oil has potent anti-fungal properties.

Maintaining Gut Health: Probiotics

Perhaps one of the most important supplements to incorporate into your anti-fungal regimen is a high-quality probiotic supplement. Probiotics, such as *Lactobacillus acidophilus*, are beneficial bacteria that live inside the terrain of the gut. They live symbiotically within our bodies performing a number of functions vital to good health; these "good" bacteria aid in energy production, produce B vitamins, aid in digestion and strengthen the immune system. Mainstream health practitioners have even become keen on the benefits provided by these bacteria, and probiotic supplements can easily be found at many groceries, convenience stores and pharmacies.

We are born with these bacteria in our systems, but over time a combination of stress, medication use, poor diet and exposure to mycotoxins, like antibiotics, alcohol or environmental toxins can deplete these cultures of good bacteria. This is one way that toxic fungal species gain a stronghold in the gut, paving the way for disease-causing fungi to proliferate and cause health problems. By reintroducing and re-colonizing these beneficial bacteria in the gut, you may be putting yourself in the best position to both prevent fungal infections and be rid of them elsewhere in the body.

As you begin to feel better and better, there are a few additional changes that you will likely want to make part of your Kaufmann Life-style. Now let's learn more about those!

CHAPTER 12

Read the Book? Check. Studied the Diet? Check. Getting Pumped? Check.

Thank you for getting this far in the book. Eleven chapters ago, the goal was to teach you about irrefutable science that links fungus to numerous health problems, a science that the medical community is largely unaware of. Now, along with your new found dietary changes and improving health, let's discuss some of the "forever tools" necessary to maintain this newfound health and further improve it at any age or stage of life. Diet alone is a very useful leg on the table, but it takes more legs to make the table sturdy.

Regardless of your improving health now, there is always room for improvement particularly if you understand the fungus link to disease. This knowledge puts the power and the responsibility of health back into your hands.

Remember, with the exception of your teeth, fungus can infect every tissue in the human body. Knowing this, a lifestyle that promotes health, beauty and wellness is necessarily one that is actively anti-fungal. I would like to outline more ways that you can remedy fungal problems and prevent exposure to these organisms and their poisons to begin with.

The Kaufmann Lifestyle

Yesterday, I went into my office and it smelled like mildew. Sure enough, I called our air condition repair company and a few hours later, they found the problem (clogged valve) and repaired it. Three hours later, my office was as fresh as new, but my lungs were not. I took a couple of garlic capsules, sprayed my nose with an anti-fungal spray, and today I feel as good as I ever have. Going back into that office day after day and not knowing why it smelled like mildew would have likely jump started my misery following my return home from Vietnam long ago. When you're aware of the damage that fungus can cause, be vigilant to minimize your exposure to it.

The basic principle of The Kaufmann lifestyle is understanding that even the smallest exposures to fungi and mycotoxins can build up over time and compromise the delicate balance in your body that keeps their harmful effects at bay. The Kaufmann Diet is a central part of that lifestyle, because gut balance is a barometer for our entire system. Researchers have discovered that 70% of our immunity lies in our guts! If the balance of good yeast and bacteria is off in our guts, it can cause the very symptoms and diseases that I have discussed in this book—and more.

This program is a lifestyle, not just a diet, because there is more to great health than what we eat. Fungi and mycotoxins gain access to our bodies in ways other than food. The air we inhale, the medications we take, the choices we make about one seemingly harmless glass of wine, might all be exposing us to fungal mycotoxins. The Kaufmann Lifestyle is all about recognizing that fungal exposures are common and making efforts to avoid them when noticed.

Your Personal Volume Switch

After 40+ years of teaching people about fungal disorders, I became a great listener, because each person I worked with brought a new set of circumstances to the table. This is likely part of the reason why most doctors do not actively address the possible fungus link to their patient's health problems. It is very time consuming. You may have read a recent publication that stated that the time our doctor has to listen to us is about 11 seconds! As you will see in our Spore Score test, it takes a lot of time to put the pieces of the fungal puzzle together for each patient. This is exactly why you need to be an active participant in your own recovery and to make your doctor a participant also.

Because I had the time to listen, I have so many of you to thank for the lessons that you taught me. In a nutshell, I learned that fungal infections could be minor or life threatening even to the point of mimicking serious diseases like diabetes and cancer. Fungus does not have an off-on switch. How I wish it did. Unless it is a brand new fungal infection or a superficial (skin) fungal problem, a pill does not readily fix it. Even if it is superficial, active surveillance is recommended. Fungus must be controlled, and depending on how long you've had it or where it is growing inside you, this takes a great deal of energy and time on your part. Many have told me that the time they spend surveilling and working on staying actively anti-fungal actually paled in comparison to time spent in so many doctors offices and pharmacies, so it is well worth your effort.

I had two musician sons and learned early in their lives about volume switches. When practicing in the house, the volume switch was 2 or 3, but on stage it was 7 or 9. When dealing with fungus, the same is true of the Kaufmann Lifestyle. Unless you have a serious, advanced disease that is responding well to the anti-fungal program, you may have the occasion to have a glass of wine with a friend or a slice of birthday cake, thereby, perhaps re-stimulating a bit of fungal activity. In essence, you're "turning up the volume" on your symptoms, if you will, to a 2 or 3. There is nothing wrong with this, as it may allow you to see a definite pattern develop. Perhaps each time you turn up the volume a bit, you experience a flare up of your symptoms, perhaps not. If so, do not crank the volume up to 7-9. If not, you may be getting better.

A Word About "Cheating" on This Program

This is a word that I purposefully avoided using in this book when it came to diet. Cheating is a bad thing, but "challenging" is not. You don't cheat when you've been on the Kaufmann 1 Diet for 6 weeks and decide you want to try a piece of mushroom pizza. If you cheat, you'd feel horrible about making such a poor decision. But by trying that pizza, you have actually challenged several foods, including wheat and mushroom, that are not on the Kaufmann 1 Diet. At 6 weeks, some people would feel absolutely nothing after challenging their system with a piece of mushroom pizza, but some would. How should that be interpreted? Well, if the symptoms return for a day or so, you know that not enough starving has taken place. So maintain the diet for another 6 weeks, and try the challenge test again, perhaps this time with a piece of dessert instead of mushroom pizza. But if that first challenge of pizza did not bring back any symptoms, this helps you evaluate your fungal problem. Perhaps it was less serious than you had thought, in that the challenge did not bring back your symptoms. Don't do what so many tend to do. Most will have another piece the next day and another the following day. I can assure you that this pattern may have you crashing by day 2 or 3 and wishing you'd have never been so aggressive. But at very least, in both cases, the challenge worked, and you are more knowledgeable because of it! If I had cancer and was improving on the diet, challenging the diet would not be in my immediate future. But if I had eczema, I might be tempted to challenge the diet somewhere along the road to recovery.

Let's face it, fungi are everywhere, and that means that we are all exposed to them on a regular basis. While our immune systems are designed to protect us against disease-causing fungi, parts of our modern lifestyle render us more vulnerable to dangerous forms of exposure than we likely would be subjected to otherwise. Let us go through the ways by which we are exposed to fungi and mycotoxins and what we can do differently.

Medicines: The Mold Is Called *Penicillium* and the Poison It Makes Is Called, *Penicillin*.

When Alexander Fleming discovered that mold limited the growth of bacteria, the world of medicine was forever changed. This discovery led to the invention of antibiotics, and while antibiotics have undoubtedly saved millions of lives, the more we used them, the more we learned. I've taught for years that antibiotics are, themselves, mycotoxins. This means that they are poisonous, as well they had better be to kill tiny living organisms like bacteria. Humans are much larger organisms, and we too have succumbed to excess antibiotic usage. Of course, the death certificate never says cause of death: antibiotics, but perhaps it should have in many cases, as you learned from slide #42 in chapter ten.

It is not the use of antibiotics that we should be concerned about, rather the abuse of them. 90 years after Fleming's discovery, a darker side of antibiotics surfaces. Antibiotic usage continues to be linked to a variety of health problems, but one notable effect is their ability to disrupt the internal gut flora. Antibiotics are indiscriminate bacteria killers; they kill both the bad bacteria causing your fever and chills, but they also kill good bacteria thereby allowing pathogenic yeasts to gain access to the gut. From there, they can proliferate throughout the body. Currently, even our Center For Disease Control (CDC) states that 33% of prescribed antibiotics are not needed.

When you live The Kaufmann Lifestyle, you become very judicious about medications prescribed to you including antibiotics. Yes, sometimes they can still be lifesaving, but the time to express your concern about antibiotics is in the doctor's office when given the prescription. Ask if your infections might be a fungal infection, and ask if you can be tested for fungus before taking a medication for bacterial infections. Tell the doctor if your home is moldy or if you were recently exposed to mold. The point is, antibiotics are now handed out by doctors like candy on Halloween. Since he won't, you must inquire about the infection he is treating. Is it really bacterial, or might it be fungus? Be nice, as doctors don't mind inquisitiveness.

Steroids, a common treatment for pain and inflammation, are another thing you must be knowledgeable of. Doctors prescribe them orally or as injections. Doctors may say that there are no side effects, but that depends on how you define a side effect. Steroids can affect our hormone functions. When we are on steroids, fungi and mycotoxins behave, well... like they are on steroids! While on steroids, you may experience more intense symptoms of any fungal-induced health problems like those discussed in this book, or you may begin to see those symptoms for the first time after taking steroids.

If you have taken steroids, or find yourself in a situation where you feel you must, taking anti-fungal supplements and sticking to The Kaufmann 1 Diet might be great ways to recover. However, with steroids you are always taking a risk that you may not recover. By taking an aggressive stance against fungal infection with your diet and anti-fungal supplements, you may reduce inflammation more naturally. Inflammation is a common immune response to invaders such as fungi. Help your body fight fungi, and it may stop producing inflammation. As you know, inflammation means swelling. If you find yourself swollen, ask yourself this simple question; what makes bread become swollen? Yeast! BINGO!

If you are starting this lifestyle for the first time, make sure you discuss this with your doctor. Some doctors will be relieved that you are not bullying them anymore for antibiotics for the common cold. Some will resist the idea that most of our sicknesses have a fungal cause. If yours is one of the later, there are a few things you can do. First, give them this book but only if they promise to really read it and return it to you. Perhaps they have never been exposed to this information. Second, you can find another doctor either for a second opinion or permanently. Inquire of the scheduling person if this new doctor treats fungal infections before you schedule. Local health food stores are a valuable resource for getting names of doctors who diagnose fungal infections. Finally, know that there are times when it really is a bacterial infection, and it makes sense to just take the antibiotic as long as you follow it up with an aggressive probiotic program. If you have been off The Kaufmann 1 Diet for example, you might try getting back on it for 30-60 days until your symptoms clear up. Most importantly through this book, you have learned that fungal mycotoxins make you vulnerable to both bacterial and fungal infections, since they suppress your immune system. This might help you to better understand that the very reason you are constantly needing an antibiotic is likely because of immune-suppressing mold in your environment, which leads us to contaminated air.

Contaminated Air

One of the benefits of modern construction is the efficiency it affords our indoor cooling and heating systems. Modern construction, however, can also provide a breeding ground for mold to flourish. Particularly in water-damaged buildings, mold can colonize in dark, unseen corners, feeding on building materials such as wood and drywall. Anywhere with a steady supply of moisture such as condensation, a leak in a roof or a broken pipe can provide a haven for mold. These mold colonies can then release spores and mycotoxins into the air, contaminating what you breathe when you are in that building.

Poor quality air remains one of the most overlooked ways by which we expose ourselves to fungi and their poisons. While researchers continue to affirm the link between indoor mold contamination and the exacerbation of allergies and/or asthma, I believe that poor indoor air may be responsible for far more than just breathing problems. It is an entry point to your body for fungi and mycotoxins, and you can end up with fungal contamination throughout your body from your nose.

With The Kaufmann Lifestyle, you understand the high importance of checking the quality of air in your home; this can reveal hidden problems that require addressing. Particularly if you are experiencing symptoms of unknown origin, testing the air in your home may reveal the hidden cause of your symptoms. Do you feel worse in your home or upon arising each morning? So often this is the case after spending an entire night inhaling mold spores from your ducting system in your home. Try an air filter near your bed for a few nights, and see if you feel better upon arising. If you do, consider getting your HVAC system cleaned. How old is your pillow? In 2005, researchers at the University of Manchester discovered millions of spores of fungus live right under our noses… in our pillows to be exact! The study pillows were 1.5 to 20 years old, and they had anywhere from 4 to 16 different molds living in them. One of the common molds was *Aspergillus fumigatus* which produces a noxious mycotoxin called, *gliotoxin*. Although *Aspergillus* may be inhaled from a pillow, in its invasive form, it can spread throughout the organs in your body including the brain. Synthetic pillows harbored more mold than natural down pillows. Replacing older pillows might be the first start if you find yourself worse upon arising.

Do-it-yourself home test kits are readily available at hardware stores. Many require being shipped off to determine exactly what species of mold is prevalent in your home. There are also a number of companies that deal with mold infestation and remediation. These companies can easily test for mold in your home and determine what level of remediation is required.

While sometimes mold infestation is obvious, other times it can lurk in homes that appear to be very clean. Particularly if your home has ever been through a flood, had a pipe break or experienced a leak that allowed rain inside, testing your home for mold contamination is a good idea, and there are many competent companies that test home air. If the testing company also offers remediation services, be careful. I'd stick with one company to test my home and another to fix my home if needed. If you have done all you can and you are still experiencing symptoms, you might just have to move to a different house or even a different climate.

The Importance of Exercise

Our bodies are designed to be strong and mobile, and there is perhaps no greater truth than the phrase, move it or lose it. We have known now for years that exercise is key for good health. Hardly a week goes by without the release of another study extolling the benefits and necessity of exercise for good health. There are reasons that I recommend exercise beyond the obvious.

Not only is exercise good for immune health, muscular health, skeletal health, cardiovascular health and mental health, it also plays a key role in your fight against disease-causing fungi. Exercising and the benefits it affords the body simply put your body in the best position to prevent a fungal infection. Exercise causes sweating, and sweating helps our bodies to detoxify heavy metals and other poisonous substances within. If you're feeling good, exercise often promotes that feeling to great! It takes several weeks to get to the point when you experience the many benefits of exercise, but getting there is worth the experience!

When you choose to live The Kaufmann Lifestyle, you exercise regularly. You know that moving your body causes it to wake any sleeping microbial giants and keeps your immune system on the alert, which plays a key role in preventing pathogenic fungi from gaining a stronghold in your body. Maximizing that immune system through exercise plays a key role in maintaining your body's natural defense mechanisms which may help prevent disease from forming in the first place. Remember, exercise can help eliminate toxins through muscle oxidation and sweating. When muscles break down, they release toxins that the body sweeps out through our pores.

Disciplining Your Thoughts

Every diet and lifestyle requires discipline which comes more naturally to some than others. If we are honest with ourselves, long term commitments to diet and exercise are extremely difficult to make. This is the part where those of us who do not like discipline roll our eyes and prepare ourselves for a battle we really do not even want to engage in. Or we enthusiastically say, I am in! Before you read this book, you had little hope of improving your health, but now you have it. Discipline is easiest when our objective is within striking distance. If the diet had you feeling better in 10 days, your hope is almost infectious. Get that home tested, buy a new pillow, exercise and maintain that diet! Watch what next month brings. In short, you can do this!

Bringing the Lifestyle and Diet Together

The Kaufmann Diet is in two distinct phases, Kaufmann 1 and Kaufmann 2. The names sometimes makes people think they are temporary. They are actually phases, because there is a bit of a transitional nature to them. Kaufmann 1 is designed for people who need an aggressive plan to starve, kill and remove fungi and mycotoxins from their bodies and to restore the good bacteria they need to maintain good gut balance. Kaufmann 2 is designed for people who have already achieved that balance.

A body in balance can fight off the stragglers that may come with Kaufmann 2 foods. However, you can live happy and healthy for the rest of your life on Kaufmann 1 alone, and I know many who have. As we mentioned in chapter eight on menopause, there are some women who do not experience the symptoms of menopause. All of the women I know who did not experience those symptoms chose to live a very healthy lifestyle, including The Kaufman 1 organic foods for many years before they began menopause. If you are close to that stage of life or already in it, you cannot turn back the clock. However, you can start a Kaufmann 1 Diet and possibly decrease the frequency and severity of your symptoms.

Your diet is a major part of how you choose to live your life. If you choose to put into your mouth only things that are beneficial to your health, you may live the rest of your life moving between Kaufmann

1 and Kaufmann 2 using your body's reactions as your indicator of when to move. If you get sick or do not feel well, you can easily back shift to Kaufmann 1. When all is well, step up to Kaufmann 2.

Some of you will feel too restricted on any diet, including The Kaufmann Diet. Now that you know what to do with symptoms, give yourself permission to challenge foods that are not on the diet every now and then. No one enjoys being around the person who talks about her diet in group gatherings. Feel free not to be that person, and eat some cake at the wedding. Do you feel worse the next day? The challenge was a huge success, because you now know to avoid cake for a longer period of time!

I typically use Thanksgiving as one of my challenge days. It is interesting, though, how I usually feel terrible the day after Thanksgiving. Experiencing this year after year has actually helped to strengthen my resolve for all other times. You may be willing to tolerate more or less than that. More than anything, now that you know where the wagon is, you can easily get back on it if you fall off. This book is always here to lend you a hand.

Congratulations! You Are Now Empowered

Before you began to read this book, you were a slave to your symptoms. You felt bad and you did not know why. Or, you have been suffering from one of the diseases we have discussed in this book. All your trips to the doctor gave no lasting relief, and you were about ready to give up hope.

What I hope I have given you in this book (and particularly in the specifics of The Kaufmann Diet and The Kaufmann Lifestyle) is a volume switch for your symptoms. When you were a slave, your symptoms turned on by themselves and increased in volume like the stereo of a rebellious teen, only you were not in control of the volume. Now you have the power to turn your symptoms down by turning the Kaufmann 1 Diet up if symptoms flare. *You are in charge of your life, because with this book and its content, you now own the volume control!* Respect and use it...

Now you know the amazing secret of this incredible, yet very credible science! Well done!

Appendix
Your Spore Score

Unbeknownst to fungi, they are not here to injure man. Of course they do, but that is not their primary purpose. Yes, they have adapted to leaning on us for a nice, warm environment and constant food supply, but until they find us, their primary job is to decompose environmental waste. Given the waste in our country alone, fungi must constantly reproduce new workers. They do this by reproducing themselves in a process called sporulation. Fungi make spores to continue their life cycle. The naked eye cannot see fungal spores, but we know that they exist, because they perform their work with great fervor.

Not only are fungi experts at reproducing themselves, but they figured out the idea of taxis long before we did. Once fungal reproduction takes place within the spore, transportation is essential. Fungal "taxi rides" take place in many ways. Birds and bugs can transport fungal spores, but for very long distance travel, spores must rely on their best friend—the wind. With new fallen trees to break down and garbage to decompose, they travel great distances to do their work.

Every physician knows that fungi are responsible for human decomposition after we die, but few know that they are also largely responsible for decomposing our bodies *before we die*. Why is that? In 1999, The World Health Organization (WHO) issued a bulletin that enables all of us who worked in the field of fungal disorders to better understand why we were witnessing such resistance to fungal diagnoses within the medical community. It stated, "*Mycotoxicoses often remain unrecognized by medical professionals, except when large numbers of people are involved.*" [1] No wonder! Medical offices see one unique patient at a time. If they saw 60 simultaneous patients who were severely bleeding and who all ate peanuts from the same bag, eventually they would figure it out.

The fact remains that people are getting better on The Kaufmann Diet and Lifestyle, yet because doctors learned very little about fungus during their medical training, the results I have achieved seem a bit sensational. I recall reading a quote from Kevin Feige around the time I began working in medical clinics and seeing hundreds of sick patients improve on my diet and anti-fungal medications: *"Rejection is common. Learning that early and often will help you build up the tolerance and resistance to keep going and keep trying."* This saying has continued to inspire me to fight the good fight.

A sad commentary on the problem of accurately diagnosing fungal symptoms and diseases was penned in an abstract published in 2004 in a journal called, *Medical Mycology*. It read, *"…the number of immunocompromised patients and subsequent invasive fungal infections continues to rise. However, the education of future medical mycologists to engage this growing problem is diminishing. While there are an increasing number of publications and grants awarded in mycology, the time and detail devoted to teaching medical mycology in United States medical schools are inadequate."* [2]

Couple this with the difficulty in testing for fungus, and it becomes painfully obvious why we have a health crisis in America. Testing a child's throat for bacteria now takes a few minutes, but testing a child's throat for fungus can take a week. Of course, since physicians learn that infections are primarily bacterial, a demand for an immediate fungal diagnostic test had never been deemed important. Although this is changing, in 2018, much remains the same.

How Do You Know If Health Problems Are Linked to Fungus?

We have discussed the problem of receiving an accurate fungal diagnosis, although there is a growing number of integrative physicians that are becoming very good at it, and I congratulate them. In all of my teachings during the past 45 years, the inevitable question always arises as to how we lay people might differentiate between fungal symptoms and those caused by bacteria or viruses. When it comes to fungus, clues are often more accurate than facts. Read that sentence again; the scientific literature is replete with articles that refer to the diagnostic problems that doctors have when trying to identify fungus as the cause of a variety of health problem.

Here is some information from an infographic that I recently prepared for educational purposes. I tried to point out that while fungi are truly the root cause of much human suffering, they often masquerade as catastrophic disorders:

Recent scientific publications state that fungal infections mimic colorectal cancer, skeletal tuberculosis, Ewing's sarcoma, bone cancer, lupus, gram-negative bacterial infection, lung cancer, thyroid mass, Alzheimer's disease, tendonitis, Crohn's disease, lacrimal sac abscess, clostridium difficile infection, osteomyelitis, chronic sinusitis.

Yes, each of these illnesses—and more—can be mimicked buy fungal infections!

Clostridium difficile? Is that not the "bacteria" that causes diarrhea? Indeed it is, but fungi can also induce diarrhea. Perhaps one day someone will redefine gram negative "bacteria" as fungi or mycotoxins. Medical education expounds on bacteriology rather than mycology for a reason, as there are hundreds of antibiotics on the market today and only a handful of anti-fungal medications. This knowledge alone tends to indoctrinate young medical students that disease-causing bacteria are a huge problem, while disease-causing fungi are not. Given this, it is important that you understand how your lifestyle might have set you up for a fungal illness, be it a local skin disorder or a deeper fungal condition that is now masquerading as a serious disease.

By no means is this questionnaire diagnostic. Based upon research concerning known fungal risk factors, the questionnaire is used to assess the degree to which you may be or have been exposed to fungi and the odds that fungi or their mycotoxins lie behind a given problem. Consider it a "ball-parker" to assist you and your doctor in accurately understanding the role that fungus might have in your health condition. This questionnaire and a careful medical history that covers questions like these can be of tremendous value to the diagnostician.

References:
(1) Peraica, M, et al. "Toxic Effects of Mycotoxins in Humans." Bulletin of the World Health Organization, vol. 77, no. 9, 1977, pp. 754–756.
(2) Steinbach, William J., et al. "Status of Medical Mycology Education." Medical Mycology, vol. 41, no. 6, 2003, pp. 457–467., doi:10.1080/13693780310001631322.

Your Spore Score

1. At any time in your life, have you taken repeated or prolonged rounds of antibiotics?

   _____

2. Are you allergic to any medications?

   _____

3. At any time in your life, have you taken repeated or prolonged courses of steroids or cortisone-based pills?

   _____

4. Do you have fingernail/toenail or scalp fungus?

   _____

5. Have you ever had ringworm or other skin problems?

   _____

6. Had you spent time in a construction site when your illness began?

   _____

7. Have you ever slept or spent time in a basement?

   _____

8. Do you have breathing problems?

   _____

9. Does your job place you underneath buildings or underground?

   _____

10. Do you suffer from dandruff?

   _____

11. Have you been diagnosed with attention deficit disorder (ADD) or hyperactivity?

_____

12. Do your bones, muscles or joints bother you?

_____

13. Do you have a chronic cough?

_____

14. Do you suffer from fatigue? Circle your energy level (10 is lowest).
    1 2 3 4 5 6 7 8 9 10

15. Do you often feel irritable?

_____

16. Do you often feel dazed or "spaced out?"

_____

17. Do you suffer from memory loss?

_____

18. Have you ever had chronic sinusitis?

_____

19. Do your ears chronically itch?

_____

20. Do you eat breakfast cereals, bread, pasta or pastries daily?

_____

21. Do you crave sugar?

_____

22. How many glasses of alcohol do you drink weekly on average?

_____

23. Have you ever been treated for parasites or worms?

_____

24. Have you been diagnosed with diabetes?

_____

25. Have you been diagnosed with cancer?

_____

26. Have you been diagnosed with migraine or hormonal headaches?

_____

27. Do you have seasonal or "all-the-time" allergies?

_____

28. Do you have high cholesterol/triglycerides?

_____

29. Are you bothered by recurring problems with your digestive tract such as bloating, belching, gas, constipation, diarrhea, abdominal pain, indigestion, or reflux?

_____

30. Have you ever been diagnosed with an autoimmune disease? Specify the disease, including when you were diagnosed.

_____

31. Do you feel worse on overcast or rainy days?

_____

32. Does your skin itch after a bath or shower?

_____

33. Have you ever been diagnosed with depression?

_____

34. Has a home you have lived in ever experienced a mold problem, or leaked? When?

_____

35. Do fabric store odors, smoke, or chemical smells bother you?

_____

36. Do you have food allergies?

_____

37. Have you been diagnosed with a neurological illness?

_____

38. Has a mammogram identified "calcification" or ductal carcinoma in-situ?

_____

39. Have you ever taken birth control pills? Did they cause complications?

_____

40. Have you ever had uterine, vaginal or urinary tract problems such as endometriosis, polycystic ovarian syndrome, UTIs or fibroids?

_____

41. Do you have fertility problems?

_____

How to Interpret This Questionnaire

Once again, know that no matter what your score on this questionnaire, you did not pass or fail. Better yet, it gives you subjective data that you have never had before that can definitely help in an accurate diagnosis. The *Spore Score* is scoreless, because there are no right or wrong answers, but it is loaded with relevant information to assist you in defining the probability that fungus or fungal mycotoxins might or might not be contributing to your health conditions.

Obviously, if you have scored a "0" on this questionnaire, it is unlikely (but not impossible) that your health conditions could be linked to fungus. Conversely, a score of 40 does not automatically implicate fungus as the cause of your health problems, although it is very likely that it is. Your *Spore Score*, therefore, must be taken in context with other factors like your age, weight, exercise program and lifestyle in order to better interpret it. The most important missing data on the questionnaire has to do with what is written on the pages of your personal doctor's office patient chart. Couple this score with the information in your medical records, and you have got some very valuable data that will help your doctor accurately diagnose your condition.

Index

Thank You

I might have written this book all alone, but I enlisted the valuable assistance of Kyle Drew and Jim Miller, both dear friends from OKC. They know about book writing and publishing, but better yet they know me and my work in the field of fungus!

THANKS, KYLE AND JIM!

About the Author
Who Is Doug Kaufmann?

1968 was a frightening time for an American 18-year-old boy. The Vietnam War was being ramped up, and we could all watch the carnage of helicopters and body bags on the 6 o'clock news each night. My friends were getting draft notices and being sent to Vietnam within months. In lieu of accepting that plight, I quickly enlisted in the U.S. Navy, where I became convinced that the very worst thing that could happen to me was to be stationed on a U.S. Navy ship somewhere near Vietnam. I could do that! Anchors away!

I served in the U.S. Navy from 1968-1974 as a hospital corpsman. I had no idea what a hospital corpsman even was, but I knew that every Navy ship had at least one of them on it, so I still felt safe! Somewhere in all of this, I learned that hospital corpsmen served in combat duty with The U.S. Marine Corps. In that capacity, I was trained in emergency medicine and served in Vietnam with the 7th Marines both in the field and at First Medical Battalion Hospital in DaNang, Vietnam. I left for Vietnam about 2 years into my six-year stint in the Navy.

I returned home to Los Angeles from Vietnam in 1971 at the age of 21. That age is relevant to my story and my discovery as you will learn.

If you have ever experienced a monsoon weather pattern like those seen in Vietnam, you know how miserable they can be. Now, imagine a monsoon weather front that lasts an entire week or two. Strong wind and drenching rain are the standard. Imagine a few more things: living outside during that week with no daylight half of the time, no walls, no heat, no change of clothes or shoes, no bathroom and knowing that people who want to kill you are hunting you. Ok, now you've got it!

Those stresses have much to do with what we Americans have called post traumatic stress disorder, or PTSD. PTSD messes with your mind, but so does neurotoxic fungus. This is where my age becomes relevant to my discovery. Recall that we stayed wet for weeks at a time without changing our clothes. This gave us the strangest rashes you had ever seen. Jungle rot, a type of fungus was common, and I had my share of it. You bring jungle rot home from Vietnam. Certain germs can enter our bodies transdermally, and I am 100% convinced that this fungus gained access to the inside of me this way.

Loud noises setting us off is a given for every combat action veteran and very understandable. But within several months of my return from Vietnam, my arms started bleeding at the folds of skin at my elbows. I began having horrible gut problems, and I began experiencing paranoia problems, especially when getting into an elevator with other people. I simply began climbing the 9 floors of stairs in the medical school I worked in upon returning home rather than ride up the elevator. But it was more complicated than just these symptoms, and that would take me some years to piece together.

Simultaneous to my having these strange symptoms was the fact that I was now 21 years old. California sets the minimum age to buy or consume alcohol at 21 years. I now realize that this formed the perfect storm! You see, our immune system can fend off fungal infections, unless we don't allow it to do its job. Fungi must have beer—lots of beer and other carbohydrates—to thrive inside our bodies. By simply combining my health related fungal problems with their favorite food (carbohydrates) I had ensured my continue suffering. Of course, what respectable 21-year-old man drinks beer without Mexican food? Soon, corn tortillas and chips and more beer ignited my health problems, and the cycle of chronic illness began.

But if diet could feed my illness, could a different diet starve it? Indeed it can! Few know that fungi are human parasites, and as such, they must eat or they will die. Without carbohydrates, like the hops, malt and barley I was consuming in beer, fungi slowly become defeated. Armed with this information in the 1970s, I began building a diet that could, in essence, literally starve fungi. This was entirely new in 1971 and unfortunately, remains new in 2019. Many popular diets are very close today, but their authors remain unaware as to how or why they actually work.

This discovery will one day change physicians' denial that diet plays a role in their patients' suffering. The good news is that many are now placing their patients on The Kaufmann 1 Diet and the results speak for themselves.

As you partake of this diet, know three things. First, if you have a medical condition and are on medication, please get your doctor's approval to follow this diet. He/she knows your medical history, and I do not. Second, deeper or very long-term fungal growth may require the use of anti-fungal medication along with this diet. If within a few weeks you are not feeling improvement on the diet, you might inquire about taking a systemic anti-fungal medication like Diflucan or Sporanox. Third and finally, give it the old college try, but know that many people experience a "healing crisis" for a few days or a period of time where they actually feel worse before they wake up a few days later feeling much better. Generally, within a week some feel better, within 2 weeks more feel better and within 4 weeks the majority of people will likely feel much better. A month on a diet cures nothing, but it serves to help you to finally understand why you have been so sick for so long. This diet can provide a wake up call to change!

Let me emphasize this final statement, because it is the platform of this entire diet and manuscript: For you or me not to fully understand this food-fungus cycle of illness is understandable. I believe it is incomprehensible, however, for those trained in medicine to not know the obvious dietary fuel link to fungal disorders. The good news is, more and more are now witnessing it, because patients like you are educating them. Like I once was, you may be suffering from a systemic fungal disorder driven by your diet and not even know it. For this reason, the book you hold in your hands could be life changing and even lifesaving. Once you experience the power of this diet, it is incumbent upon you to share it with the doctors who doubted and with your loved ones. Thank you in advance!

– Doug Kaufmann, 2018